Health Care Essentials

Health Care Essentials

Editor: Ronald Tripp

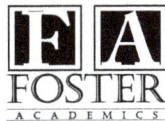

FA **FOSTER**
A C A D E M I C S

www.fosteracademics.com

www.fosteracademics.com

FA
FOSTER
ACADEMICS

Cataloging-in-Publication Data

Health care essentials / edited by Ronald Tripp.
    p. cm.
Includes bibliographical references and index.
ISBN 978-1-63242-545-4
1. Medical care. 2. Public health. I. Tripp, Ronald.
RA411 .H43 2018
362.1--dc23

Foster Academics,
118-35 Queens Blvd., Suite 400,
Forest Hills, NY 11375, USA

ISBN 978-1-63242-545-4 (Hardback)

Contents

Permissions

Index

Health care refers to the maintenance, development and improvement of health care facilities. It includes the study of treatments, prevention, diagnosis and cure of diseases and illnesses that plague the earth and affect human beings. There are many professions that come under this vast field namely physicians, dentists, doctors, surgeons, allied health professionals, etc. This book is compiled in such a manner, that it will provide in-depth knowledge about the theories of health care. Also included in it is a detailed explanation of the various concepts and applications of the subject. The textbook is appropriate for those seeking detailed information in this area.

A foreword of all Chapters of the book is provided below:

Chapter 1 - The act of taking necessary measures for the prevention, treatment and diagnosis of diseases in human beings is known as health care. It can be divided into primary care, secondary care and tertiary care. This chapter has been carefully written to provide an easy understanding of the varied facets of health care; **Chapter 2 -** Health facilities can be of various types like health care centers, hospitals, medical nursing homes, pharmacies and drug stores, etc. These facilities can be owned by individuals or governments. The chapter on health care facilities offers an insightful focus, keeping in mind the complex subject matter; **Chapter 3 -** Health administration is the management of hospitals, health care systems and public health systems. Hospital administrators may be generalists or specialists. Health care management is best understood in confluence with the major topics listed in the following section; **Chapter 4 -** A group of people or institutions that focus on meeting the demands of health care are a part of the health system. Universal health care is a health care system in which a country's citizens are promised medical aid as well as financial guarantee. The aspects elucidated in this chapter are of vital importance, and provide a better understanding of health care.

I would like to thank the entire editorial team who made sincere efforts for this book and my family who supported me in my efforts of working on this book. I take this opportunity to thank all those who have been a guiding force throughout my life.

Editor

Understanding Health Care

The act of taking necessary measures for the prevention, treatment and diagnosis of diseases in human beings is known as health care. It can be divided into primary care, secondary care and tertiary care. This chapter has been carefully written to provide an easy understanding of the varied facets of health care.

Health Care

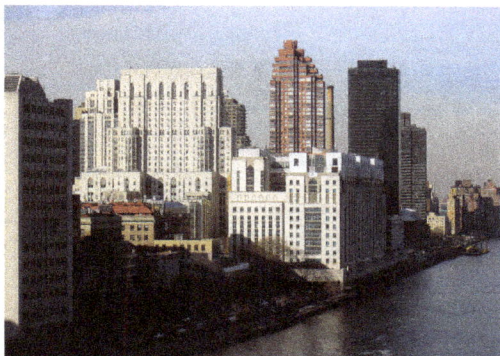

New York-Presbyterian Hospital in New York City is one of the world's busiest hospitals. Pictured is the Weill-Cornell facility (white complex at centre).

Health care or healthcare is the maintenance or improvement of health via the diagnosis, treatment, and prevention of disease, illness, injury, and other physical and mental impairments in human beings. Healthcare is delivered by health professionals (providers or practitioners) in allied health professions, chiropractic, physicians, physician associates, dentistry, midwifery, nursing, medicine, optometry, pharmacy, psychology, and other health professions. It includes the work done in providing primary care, secondary care, and tertiary care, as well as in public health.

Access to healthcare varies across countries, groups, and individuals, largely influenced by social and economic conditions as well as the health policies in place. Countries and jurisdictions have different policies and plans in relation to the personal and population-based health care goals within their societies. Healthcare systems are organizations established to meet the health needs of target populations. Their exact configuration varies between national and subnational entities. In some countries and jurisdictions, healthcare planning is distributed among market participants, whereas in others, planning occurs more centrally among governments or other coordinating bodies. In all cases, according to the World Health Organization (WHO), a well-functioning healthcare system requires a robust financing mechanism; a well-trained and adequately-paid workforce; reliable information on which to base decisions and policies; and well maintained health facilities and logistics to deliver quality medicines and technologies.

Healthcare can contribute to a significant part of a country's economy. In 2011, the healthcare industry consumed an average of 9.3 percent of the GDP or US$ 3,322 (PPP-adjusted) per capita across the 34 members of OECD countries. The USA (17.7%, or US$ PPP 8,508), the Netherlands (11.9%, 5,099), France (11.6%, 4,118), Germany (11.3%, 4,495), Canada (11.2%, 5669), and Switzerland (11%, 5,634) were the top spenders, however life expectancy in total population at birth was highest in Switzerland (82.8 years), Japan and Italy (82.7), Spain and Iceland (82.4), France (82.2) and Australia (82.0), while OECD's average exceeds 80 years for the first time ever in 2011: 80.1 years, a gain of 10 years since 1970. The USA (78.7 years) ranges only on place 26 among the 34 OECD member countries, but has the highest costs by far. All OECD countries have achieved universal (or almost universal) health coverage, except Mexico and the USA.

Healthcare is conventionally regarded as an important determinant in promoting the general physical and mental health and well-being of people around the world. An example of this was the worldwide eradication of smallpox in 1980, declared by the WHO as the first disease in human history to be completely eliminated by deliberate health care interventions.

Delivery

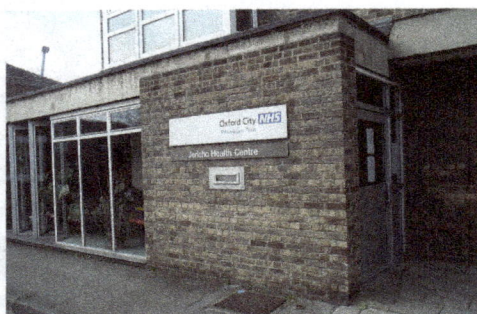

Primary care may be provided in community health centres.

The delivery of modern health care depends on groups of trained professionals and paraprofessionals coming together as interdisciplinary teams. This includes professionals in medicine, psychology, physiotherapy, nursing, dentistry, midwifery and allied health, plus many others such as public health practitioners, community health workers and assistive personnel, who systematically provide personal and population-based preventive, curative and rehabilitative care services.

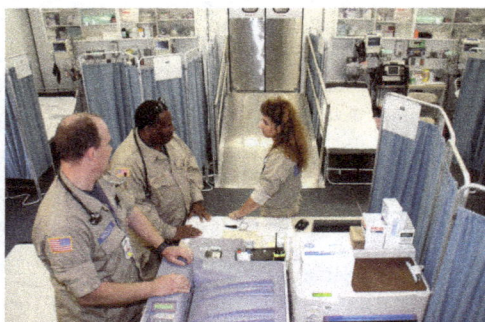

The emergency room is often a frontline venue for the delivery of primary medical care.

While the definitions of the various types of health care vary depending on the different cultural, political, organizational and disciplinary perspectives, there appears to be some consensus that primary care constitutes the first element of a continuing health care process, that may also include the provision of secondary and tertiary levels of care. Healthcare can be defined as either public or private.

Primary Care

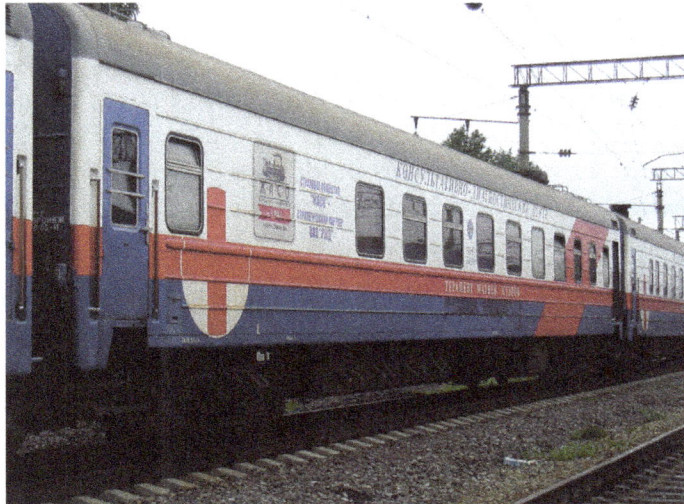

Medical train "Therapist Matvei Mudrov" in Khabarovsk, Russia

Primary care refers to the work of health professionals who act as a first point of consultation for all patients within the health care system. Such a professional would usually be a primary care physician, such as a general practitioner or family physician, a licensed independent practitioner such as a physiotherapist, or a non-physician primary care provider (mid-level provider) such as a physician assistant or nurse practitioner. Depending on the locality, health system organization, and sometimes at the patient's discretion, they may see another health care professional first, such as a pharmacist, a nurse (such as in the United Kingdom), a clinical officer (such as in parts of Africa), or an Ayurvedic or other traditional medicine professional (such as in parts of Asia). Depending on the nature of the health condition, patients may then be referred for secondary or tertiary care.

Primary care is often used as the term for the health care services which play a role in the local community. It can be provided in different settings, such as Urgent care centres which provide services to patients same day with appointment or walk-in bases.

Primary care involves the widest scope of health care, including all ages of patients, patients of all socioeconomic and geographic origins, patients seeking to maintain optimal health, and patients with all manner of acute and chronic physical, mental and social health issues, including multiple chronic diseases. Consequently, a primary care practitioner must possess a wide breadth of knowledge in many areas. Continuity is a key characteristic of primary care, as patients usually prefer to consult the same practitioner for routine check-ups and preventive care, health education, and every time they require an initial consultation about a new health problem. The International Classification of Primary Care (ICPC) is a standardized tool for understanding and analyzing information on interventions in primary care by the reason for the patient visit.

Common chronic illnesses usually treated in primary care may include, for example: hypertension, diabetes, asthma, COPD, depression and anxiety, back pain, arthritis or thyroid dysfunction. Primary care also includes many basic maternal and child health care services, such as family planning services and vaccinations. In the United States, the 2013 National Health Interview Survey found that skin disorders (42.7%), osteoarthritis and joint disorders (33.6%), back problems (23.9%), disorders of lipid metabolism (22.4%), and upper respiratory tract disease (22.1%, excluding asthma) were the most common reasons for accessing a physician.

In the United States, primary care physicians have begun to deliver primary care outside of the managed care (insurance-billing) system through direct primary care which is a subset of the more familiar concierge medicine. Physicians in this model bill patients directly for services, either on a pre-paid monthly, quarterly, or annual basis, or bill for each service in the office. Examples of direct primary care practices include Foundation Health in Colorado and Qliance in Washington.

In context of global population aging, with increasing numbers of older adults at greater risk of chronic non-communicable diseases, rapidly increasing demand for primary care services is expected in both developed and developing countries. The World Health Organization attributes the provision of essential primary care as an integral component of an inclusive primary health care strategy.

Secondary Care

Secondary care includes acute care: necessary treatment for a short period of time for a brief but serious illness, injury or other health condition, such as in a hospital emergency department. It also includes skilled attendance during childbirth, intensive care, and medical imaging services.

The term "secondary care" is sometimes used synonymously with "hospital care". However, many secondary care providers do not necessarily work in hospitals, such as psychiatrists, clinical psychologists, occupational therapists, most dental specialties or physiotherapists (physiotherapists are also primary care providers, and a referral is not required to see a physiotherapist), and some primary care services are delivered within hospitals. Depending on the organization and policies of the national health system, patients may be required to see a primary care provider for a referral before they can access secondary care.

For example, in the United States, which operates under a mixed market health care system, some physicians might voluntarily limit their practice to secondary care by requiring patients to see a primary care provider first, or this restriction may be imposed under the terms of the payment agreements in private or group health insurance plans. In other cases medical specialists may see patients without a referral, and patients may decide whether self-referral is preferred.

In the United Kingdom and Canada, patient self-referral to a medical specialist for secondary care is rare as prior referral from another physician (either a primary care physician or another specialist) is considered necessary, regardless of whether the funding is from private insurance schemes or national health insurance.

Allied health professionals, such as physical therapists, respiratory therapists, occupational therapists, speech therapists, and dietitians, also generally work in secondary care, accessed through either patient self-referral or through physician referral.

Tertiary Care

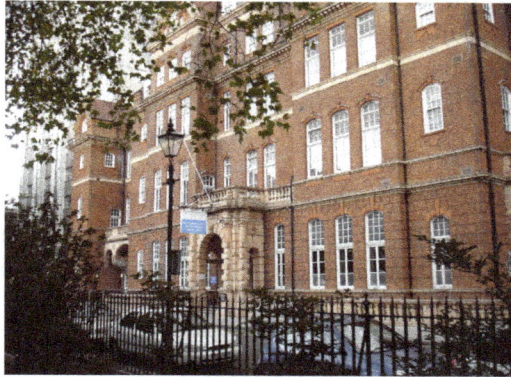

The National Hospital for Neurology and Neurosurgery in London,
United Kingdom is a specialist neurological hospital.

Tertiary care is specialized consultative health care, usually for inpatients and on referral from a primary or secondary health professional, in a facility that has personnel and facilities for advanced medical investigation and treatment, such as a tertiary referral hospital.

Examples of tertiary care services are cancer management, neurosurgery, cardiac surgery, plastic surgery, treatment for severe burns, advanced neonatology services, palliative, and other complex medical and surgical interventions.

Quaternary Care

The term quaternary care is sometimes used as an extension of tertiary care in reference to advanced levels of medicine which are highly specialized and not widely accessed. Experimental medicine and some types of uncommon diagnostic or surgical procedures are considered quaternary care. These services are usually only offered in a limited number of regional or national health care centres. This term is more prevalent in the United Kingdom, but just as applicable in the United States. A quaternary care hospital may have virtually any procedure available, whereas a tertiary care facility may not offer a sub-specialist with that training.

Home and Community Care

Many types of health care interventions are delivered outside of health facilities. They include many interventions of public health interest, such as food safety surveillance, distribution of condoms and needle-exchange programmes for the prevention of transmissible diseases.

They also include the services of professionals in residential and community settings in support of self care, home care, long-term care, assisted living, treatment for substance use disorders and other types of health and social care services.

Community rehabilitation services can assist with mobility and independence after loss of limbs or loss of function. This can include prosthesis, orthotics or wheelchairs.

Many countries, especially in the west are dealing with aging populations, and one of the priorities of the health care system is to help seniors live full, independent lives in the comfort of their own homes. There is an entire section of health care geared to providing seniors with help in day-to-day activities at home, transporting them to doctor's appointments, and many other activities that are so essential for their health and well-being. Although they provide home care for older adults in cooperation, family members and care workers may harbor diverging attitudes and values towards their joint efforts. This state of affairs presents a challenge for the design of ICT for home care.

With obesity in children rapidly becoming a major concern, health services often set up programs in schools aimed at educating children in good eating habits; making physical education compulsory in school; and teaching young adolescents to have positive self-image.

Rating s

Health care ratings are ratings or evaluations of health care used to evaluate process of care, healthcare structures and/or outcomes of a healthcare services. This information is translated into report cards that are generated by quality organizations, nonprofit, consumer groups and media. This evaluation of quality can be based on:

- Measures of Hospital quality

- Measures of Health Plan Quality

- Measures of Physician Quality

- Measures of Quality for Other Health Professionals

- Measures of Patient Experience

Related Sectors

Health care extends beyond the delivery of services to patients, encompassing many related sectors, and set within a bigger picture of financing and governance structures.

Health System

A health system, also sometimes referred to as health care system or healthcare system is the organization of people, institutions, and resources to deliver health care services to meet the health needs of target populations.

Health Care Industry

The health care industry incorporates several sectors that are dedicated to providing health care services and products. As a basic framework for defining the sector, the United Nations' International Standard Industrial Classification categorizes health care as generally consisting of hospital activities, medical and dental practice activities, and "other human health activities". The last class involves activities of, or under the supervision of, nurses, midwives, physiotherapists, scientific or diagnostic laboratories, pathology clinics, residential health facilities, patient advocates, or other allied health professions, e.g. in the field of optometry, hydrotherapy, medical massage, yoga therapy, music therapy, occupational therapy, speech therapy, chiropody, homeopathy, chiropractics, acupuncture, etc.

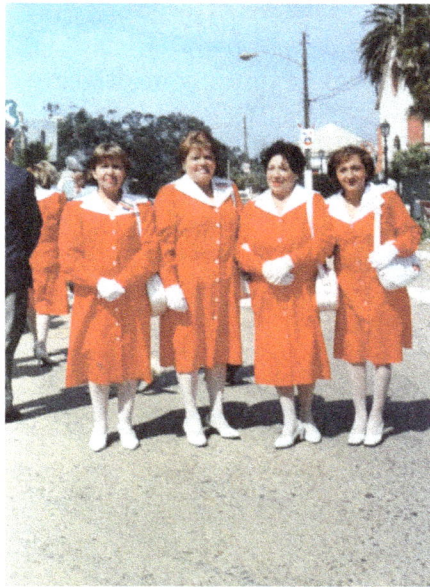

A group of Chilean 'Damas de Rojo' volunteering at their local hospital

In addition, according to industry and market classifications, such as the Global Industry Classification Standard and the Industry Classification Benchmark, health care includes many categories of medical equipment, instruments and services as well as biotechnology, diagnostic laboratories and substances, and drug manufacturing and delivery.

For example, pharmaceuticals and other medical devices are the leading high technology exports of Europe and the United States. The United States dominates the biopharmaceutical field, accounting for three-quarters of the world's biotechnology revenues.

Health Care Research

The quantity and quality of many health care interventions are improved through the results of science, such as advanced through the medical model of health which focuses on the eradication of illness through diagnosis and effective treatment. Many important advances have been made through health research, including biomedical research and pharmaceutical research, which form the basis for evidence-based medicine and evidence-based practice in health care delivery.

For example, in terms of pharmaceutical research and development spending, Europe spends a little less than the United States (€22.50bn compared to €27.05bn in 2006). The United States accounts for 80% of the world's research and development spending in biotechnology.

In addition, the results of health services research can lead to greater efficiency and equitable delivery of health care interventions, as advanced through the social model of health and disability, which emphasizes the societal changes that can be made to make population healthier. Results from health services research often form the basis of evidence-based policy in health care systems. Health services research is also aided by initiatives in the field of AI for the development of systems of health assessment that are clinically useful, timely, sensitive to change, culturally sensitive, low burden, low cost, involving for the patient and built into standard procedures.

Health Care Financing

There are generally five primary methods of funding health care systems:

1. general taxation to the state, county or municipality

2. social health insurance

3. voluntary or private health insurance

4. out-of-pocket payments

5. donations to health charities

In most countries, the financing of health care services features a mix of all five models, but the exact distribution varies across countries and over time within countries. In all countries and jurisdictions, there are many topics in the politics and evidence that can influence the decision of a government, private sector business or other group to adopt a specific health policy regarding the financing structure.

For example, social health insurance is where a nation's entire population is eligible for health care coverage, and this coverage and the services provided are regulated. In almost every jurisdiction with a government-funded health care system, a parallel private, and usually for-profit, system is allowed to operate. [1] This is sometimes referred to as two-tier health care or universal health care.

For example, in Poland, the costs of health services borne by the National Health Fund (financed by all citizens that pay health insurance contributions) in 2012 amounted to 60.8 billion PLN (approximately 20 billion USD). The right to health services in Poland is granted to 99.9% of the population (also registered unemployed persons and their spouses).

Health Care Administration and Regulation

The management and administration of health care is another sector vital to the delivery of health care services. In particular, the practice of health professionals and operation of health care institutions is typically regulated by national or state/provincial authorities through appropriate regulatory bodies for purposes of quality assurance. Most countries have credentialing staff in regulatory boards or health departments who document the certification or licensing of health workers and their work history.

Health Information Technology

Health information technology (HIT) is "the application of information processing involving both computer hardware and software that deals with the storage, retrieval, sharing, and use of health care information, data, and knowledge for communication and decision making." Technology is a broad concept that deals with a species' usage and knowledge of tools and crafts, and how it affects a species' ability to control and adapt to its environment. However, a strict definition is elusive; "technology" can refer to material objects of use to humanity, such as machines, hardware or utensils, but can also encompass broader themes, including systems, methods of organization, and techniques. For HIT, technology represents computers and communications attributes that can be networked to build systems for moving health information. Informatics is yet another integral aspect of HIT.

Health information technology can be divided into further components like Electronic Health Record (EHR), Electronic Medical Record (EMR), Personal Health Record (PHR), Practice Management System (PMS), Health Information Exchange (HIE) and many more. There are multiple purposes for the use of HIT within the health care industry. Further, the use of HIT is expected to improve the quality of health care, reduce medical errors, improve the health care service efficiency and reduce health care costs.

Primary Care

Primary care is the day-to-day healthcare given by a health care provider. Typically this provider acts as the first contact and principal point of continuing care for patients within a healthcare system, and coordinates other specialist care that the patient may need. Patients commonly receive primary care from professionals such as a primary care physician (general practitioner or family physician), a nurse practitioner (adult-gerontology nurse practitioner, family nurse practitioner, or pediatric nurse practitioner), or a physician assistant. In some localities such a professional may be a registered nurse, a pharmacist, a clinical officer (as in parts of Africa), or a Ayurvedic or other traditional medicine professional (as in parts of Asia). Depending on the nature of the health condition, patients may then be referred for secondary or tertiary care.

Background

The World Health Organization attributes the provision of essential primary care as an integral component of an inclusive primary healthcare strategy. Primary care involves the widest scope of healthcare, including all ages of patients, patients of all socioeconomic and geographic origins, patients seeking to maintain optimal health, and patients with all manner of acute and chronic physical, mental and social health issues, including multiple chronic diseases. Consequently, a primary care practitioner must possess a wide breadth of knowledge in many areas. Continuity is a key characteristic of primary care, as patients usually prefer to consult the same practitioner for routine check-ups and preventive care, health education, and every time they require an initial consultation about a new health problem. Collaboration among providers is a desirable characteristic of primary care.

The International Classification of Primary Care (ICPC) is a standardized tool for understanding and analyzing information on interventions in primary care by the reason for the patient visit. Common chronic illnesses usually treated in primary care may include, for example: hypertension, angina, diabetes, asthma, COPD, depression and anxiety, back pain, arthritis or thyroid dysfunction. Primary care also includes many basic maternal and child health care services, such as family planning services and vaccinations.

In context of global population ageing, with increasing numbers of older adults at greater risk of chonic non-communicable diseases, rapidly increasing demand for primary care services is expected around the world, in both developed and developing countries.

Primary Care by Country

United Kingdom

In the United Kingdom, patients can access primary care services through their local general practice, community pharmacy, optometrist, dental surgery and community hearing care providers. Services are generally provided free-of-charge through the National Health Service. In the UK, unlike many other countries, patients do not normally have direct access to hospital consultants and the GP controls access to secondary care. This practice is referred to as "gatekeeping"; the future of this role has been questioned by researchers who conclude *"Gatekeeping policies should be revisited to accommodate the government's aim to modernise the NHS in terms of giving patients more choice and facilitate more collaborative work between GPs and specialists. At the same time, any relaxation of gatekeeping should be carefully evaluated to ensure the clinical and non-clinical benefits outweigh the costs"*.

599 GP practices closed between 2010–11 and 2014–15, while 91 opened and average practice list size increased from 6,610 to 7,171.

According to the Local Government Association 57 million GP consultations in England in 2015 were for minor conditions and illnesses, 5.2 million of them for blocked noses.

Canada

In Canada, access to primary and other healthcare services are guaranteed for all citizens through the Canada Health Act.

Nigeria

In Nigeria, healthcare is a concurrent responsibility of three tiers of government. Local governments focus on the delivery of primary care (e.g. through a system of dispensaries), state governments manage the various general hospitals (secondary care), while the federal government's role is mostly limited to coordinating the affairs of the Federal Medical Centres and university teaching hospitals (tertiary care).

United States

A 2009 report by the New England Healthcare Institute determined that an increased demand on primary care by older, sicker patients and decreased supply of primary care practitioners has led to a crisis in primary care delivery. The research identified a set of innovations that could enhance the quality, efficiency and effectiveness of primary care in the United States.

On March 23, 2010 President Obama signed the Patient Protection and Affordable Care Act (ACA) into law. The law is expected to expand health insurance coverage by 32 million people by 2016 and 34 million people by 2021. The success of the expansion of health insurance under the ACA in large measure depends on the availability of primary care physicians. Unfortunately, The ACA has drastically exacerbated the projected deficit of primary care physicians needed to ensure care for insured Americans. According to the Association of American Medical Colleges (AAMC) without the ACA, the United States would have been short roughly 64,000 physicians by 2020; with the implementation of the ACA, it will be 91,000 physicians short. According to the AAMC's November 2009 physician work force report, nationally, the rate of physicians providing primary care is 79.4 physicians per 100,000 residents.

Primary healthcare results in better health outcomes, reduced health disparities and lower spending, including on avoidable emergency room visits and hospital care. With that being said, primary care physicians are an important component in ensuring that the healthcare system as a whole is sustainable. However, despite their importance to the healthcare system, the primary care position has suffered in terms of its prestige in part due to the differences in salary when compared to doctors that decide to specialize. In a 2010 national study of physician wages conducted by the UC Davis Health System found that specialists are paid as much as 52 percent more than primary care physicians, even though primary care physicians see far more patients.

Primary care physicians earn $60.48 per hour; specialists on average earn $88.34. A follow up study conducted by the UC Davis Health System found that earnings over the course of the careers of primary care physicians averaged as much as $2.8 million less than the earnings of their specialist colleagues. This discrepancy in pay has potentially made primary care a less attractive choice for medical school graduates. In 2011, about 17,000 doctors graduated from American medical schools and only 7 percent of graduates chose a career in primary care. The average age of a primary care physician in the United States is 47 years old, and one quarter of all primary care physicians are nearing retirement. Fifty years ago roughly half of the physicians in America practiced primary care; today, fewer than one third of them do.

US Strategies to Address the Primary Care Shortage

The Patient Protection Affordable Care Act contains a number of provisions to increase primary care capacity. These provisions are directed towards medical school graduates and include payment reform, student loan forgiveness programs and increased primary care residency positions The PPACA also provides funding and mandates to increase the role of physician extenders like nurse practitioners and physician assistants to enhance the primary care workforce. The PPCA is projected to increase patient demand for primary care services. Through the adoption of new patient care delivery models that include physicians working in tandem with nurse practitioners and physician assistants, demand for future primary care services could be met. Consumer surveys have found the American public to be open to a greater role for physician extenders in the primary care setting. Policies and laws, primarily at the state level, would need to redefine and reallocate the roles and responsibilities for non-physician licensed providers to optimize these new models of care.

Primary Healthcare

Primary healthcare (PHC) refers to "essential health care" that is based on scientifically sound and socially acceptable methods and technology, which make universal health care accessible to all individuals and families in a community. It is through their full participation and at a cost that the community and the country can afford to maintain at every stage of their development in the spirit of self-reliance and self-determination". In other words, PHC is an approach to health beyond the traditional health care system that focuses on health equity-producing social policy. PHC includes all areas that play a role in health, such as access to health services, environment and lifestyle. Thus, primary healthcare and public health measures, taken together, may be considered as the cornerstones of universal health systems.

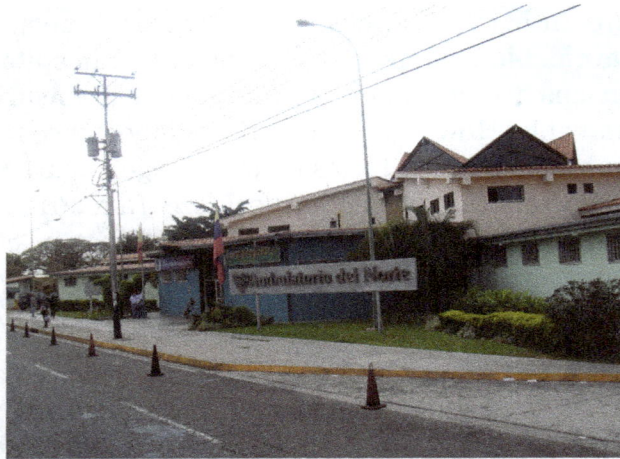

Public ambulatory care facility in Maracay, Venezuela, providing primary care for ambulatory care sensitive conditions.

This ideal model of healthcare was adopted in the declaration of the International Conference on Primary Health Care held in Alma Ata, Kazakhstan in 1978 (known as the "Alma Ata Declaration"), and became a core concept of the World Health Organization's goal of *Health for all*. The Alma-Ata Conference mobilized a "Primary Health Care movement" of professionals and institutions, governments and civil society organizations, researchers and grassroots organizations that undertook to tackle the "politically, socially and economically unacceptable" health inequalities in all countries. There were many factors that inspired PHC; a prominent example is the Barefoot doctors of China.

Goals and Principles

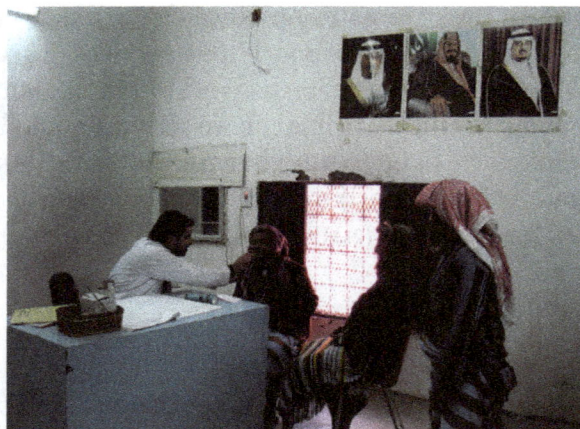

A primary health care worker in Saudi Arabia, 2008

The ultimate goal of primary healthcare is the attainment of better health services for all. It is for this reason that World Health Organization (WHO), has identified five key elements to achieving this goal:

- reducing exclusion and social disparities in health (universal coverage reforms);

- organizing health services around people's needs and expectations (service delivery reforms);

- integrating health into all sectors (public policy reforms);

- pursuing collaborative models of policy dialogue (leadership reforms); and

- increasing stakeholder participation.

Behind these elements lies a series of basic principles identified in the Alma Ata Declaration that should be formulated in national policies in order to launch and sustain PHC as part of a comprehensive health system and in coordination with other sectors:

- Equitable distribution of health care – according to this principle, primary care and other services to meet the main health problems in a community must be provided equally to all individuals irrespective of their gender, age, caste, color, urban/rural location and social class.

- Community participation – in order to make the fullest use of local, national and other available resources. Community participation was considered sustainable due to its grass roots nature and emphasis on self-sufficiency, as opposed to targeted (or vertical) approaches dependent on international development assistance.

- Health workforce development – comprehensive healthcare relies on adequate number and distribution of trained physicians, nurses, allied health professions, community health workers and others working as a health team and supported at the local and referral levels.

- Use of appropriate technology – medical technology should be provided that is accessible, affordable, feasible and culturally acceptable to the community. Examples of appropriate technology include refrigerators for vaccine cold storage. Less appropriate could include, in many settings, body scanners or heart-lung machines, which benefit only a small minority concentrated in urban areas. They are generally not accessible to the poor, but draw a large share of resources.

- Multi-sectional approach – recognition that health cannot be improved by intervention within just the formal health sector; other sectors are equally important in promoting the health and self-reliance of communities. These sectors include, at least: agriculture (e.g. food security); education; communication (e.g. concerning prevailing health problems and the methods of preventing and controlling them); housing; public works (e.g. ensuring an adequate supply of safe water and basic sanitation); rural development; industry; community organizations (including Panchayats or local governments, voluntary organizations, etc.).

In sum, PHC recognizes that healthcare is not a short-lived intervention, but an ongoing process of improving people's lives and alleviating the underlying socioeconomic conditions that contribute to poor health. The principles link health and development, advocating political interventions, rather than passive acceptance of economic conditions.

Approaches

The hospital ship USNS *Mercy* (T-AH-19) in Manado, Indonesia, during Pacific Partnership 2012.

The primary health care approach has seen significant gains in health were applied even when adverse economic and political conditions prevail.

Although the declaration made at the Alma-Ata conference deemed to be convincing and plausible in specifying goals to PHC and achieving more effective strategies, it generated numerous criticisms and reactions worldwide. Many argued the declaration did not have clear targets, was too broad, and was not attainable because of the costs and aid needed. As a result, PHC approaches have evolved in different contexts to account for disparities in resources and local priority health problems; this is alternatively called the Selective Primary Health Care (SPHC) approach.

Selective PHC

After the year 1978 Alta Alma Conference, the Rockefeller Foundation held a conference in 1979 at its Bellagio conference center in Italy to address several concerns. Here, the idea of Selective Primary Health Care was introduced as a strategy to complement comprehensive PHC. It was based on a paper by Julia Walsh and Kenneth S. Warren entitled "Selective Primary Health Care, an Interim Strategy for Disease Control in Developing Countries". This new framework advocated a more economically feasible approach to PHC by only targeting specific areas of health, and choosing the most effective treatment plan in terms of cost and effectiveness. One of the foremost examples of SPHC is "GOBI" (growth monitoring, oral rehydration, breastfeeding, and immunization), focusing on combating the main diseases in developing nations.

GOBI-FFF

Selective PHC approach consists of techniques known collectively under the acronym "GOBI-FFF". It focuses on severe population health problems in certain developing countries, where a few diseases are responsible for high rates of infant and child mortality. Health care planning is employed to see which diseases require most attention and, subsequently, which intervention can be most effectively applied as part of primary care in a least-cost method. The targets and effects of Selective PHC are specific and measurable. The approach aims to prevent most health and nutrition problems before they begin:

- Growth monitoring: the monitoring of how much infants grow within a period, with the goal to understand needs for better early nutrition.
- Oral rehydration therapy: to combat dehydration associated with diarrhea
- Breastfeeding
- Immunization
- Family planning (birth spacing)
- Female education
- Food supplementation: for example, iron and folic acid fortification/supplementation to prevent deficiencies in pregnant women.

PHC and Population Aging

Given global demographic trends, with the numbers of people age 60 and over expected to double by 2025, PHC approaches have taken into account the need for countries to address the consequences of population ageing. In particular, in the future the majority of older people will be living in developing countries that are often the least prepared to confront the challenges of rapidly ageing societies, including high risk of having at least one chronic non-communicable disease, such as diabetes and osteoporosis. According to WHO, dealing with this increasing burden requires health promotion and disease prevention intervention at community level as well as disease management strategies within health care systems.

PHC and Mental Health

Some jurisdictions apply PHC principles in planning and managing their healthcare services for the detection, diagnosis and treatment of common mental health conditions at local clinics, and organizing the referral of more complicated mental health problems to more appropriate levels of mental health care.

Background and Controversies

Barefoot Doctors

The "Barefoot doctors" of China were an important inspiration for PHC because they illustrated the effectiveness of having a healthcare professional at the community level with community ties. Barefoot doctors were a diverse array of village health workers who lived in rural areas and received basic healthcare training. They stressed rural rather than urban healthcare, and preventive rather than curative services. They also provided a combination of western and traditional medicines. They had close community ties, were relatively low-cost, and perhaps most importantly they encouraged self-reliance through advocating prevention and hygiene practices. The program experienced a massive expansion of rural medical services in China, with the number of barefoot doctors increasing dramatically between the early 1960s and the Cultural Revolution (1964-1976).

Criticisms

Although many countries were keen on the idea of primary healthcare after the Alma Ata conference, the Declaration itself was criticized for being too "idealistic" and "having an unrealistic time table". More specific approaches to prevent and control diseases - based on evidence of prevalence, morbidity, mortality and feasibility of control (cost-effectiveness) - were subsequently proposed. The best known model was the Selective PHC approach (described above). Selective PHC favoured short-term goals and targeted health investment, but it did not address the social causes of disease. As such, the SPHC approach has been criticized as not following Alma Ata's core principle of everyone's entitlement to healthcare and health system development.

In Africa, the PHC system has been extended into isolated rural areas through construction of health posts and centers that offer basic maternal-child health, immunization, nutrition, first aid, and referral services. Implementation of PHC is said to be affected after the introduction of structural adjustment programs by the World Bank.

References

- Bentley, JM; Nash, DB (1998). "How Pennsylvania hospitals have responded to publicly released reports on coronary artery bypass graft surgery?.". The Joint Commission Journal on Quality Improvement. 24 (1): 40–9

- Braveman, Paula; E. Tarimo (1994). Screening in Primary Health Care: Setting Priorities With Limited Resources. World Health Organization. p. 14. ISBN 9241544732. Retrieved 4 November 2012

- Greenfield, Geva; Foley, Kimberley; Majeed, Azeem (23 September 2016). "Rethinking primary care's gatekeeper role". BMJ: i4803. doi:10.1136/bmj.i4803

- Lagu, T.; Lindenauer, P. K. (2010). "Putting the public back in public reporting of health care quality". JAMA: The Journal of the American Medical Association. 304 (15): 1711–1712. doi:10.1001/jama.2010.1499

- Kaiser Family Foundation. "Kaiser Family Foundation and Agency for 2008 Update on Consumers' Views of Patient Safety and Quality Information" (PDF). . Retrieved February 18, 2011

- Sommers, B.D. (2012). "New physicians, the affordable care act, and the changing practice of medicine.". JAMA. 307: 1697–98. doi:10.1001/jama.2012.523

- "The effectiveness of CAHPS among women enrolling in Medicaid managed care". Journal of Ambulatory Care Management. 24 (4): 76–91. 2001. doi:10.1097/00004479-200110000-00006

- Madison, Kristen. "The Law and Policy of Health Care Quality Reporting" (PDF). Campbell Law Review. Campbell University. Retrieved March 8, 2011

- Bodenheimer, T.S. (2013). "Proposed Solutions to the physcian shortage without training more physicians". Health Affairs (Project Hope). 32: 1881–1886. doi:10.1377/hlthaff.2013.0234

- Fox, Susannah. "Peer-to-peer Healthcare". Pew Research Center's Internet & American Life Project. Pew Research Center. Retrieved March 8, 2013

2

Health Care Facilities: A Comprehensive Study

Health facilities can be of various types like health care centers, hospitals, medical nursing homes, pharmacies and drug stores, etc. These facilities can be owned by individuals or governments. The chapter on health care facilities offers an insightful focus, keeping in mind the complex subject matter.

Health Facility

Hartford Hospital in Hartford, Connecticut. A hospital is one common type of health facility.

A health facility is, in general, any location where healthcare is provided. Health facilities range from small clinics and doctor's offices to urgent care centers and large hospitals with elaborate emergency rooms and trauma centers. The number and quality of health facilities in a country or region is one common measure of that area's prosperity and quality of life. In many countries, health facilities are regulated to some extent by law; licensing by a regulatory agency is often required before a facility may open for business. Health facilities may be owned and operated by for-profit businesses, non-profit organizations, governments, and in some cases by individuals, with proportions varying by country.

Health Facility Workload

The workload of a health facility is often used to indicate its size. Large health facilities are those with a greater patient load.

In Australia the workload of a health facility is used to determine the level of government funding provided to that facility. The government measures a facility (or health practice) in terms of its standard whole patient equivalent (SWPE). The SWPE calculation is determined by analysis of the patients that attend that facility. The calculation takes into account the proportion of health services (in dollars) rendered at that facility relative to others that each patient attends. It includes a weighting factor based on each patients demography to account for the varied levels of services required by patients depending on their gender and age. The premise of weighting is that patients require different levels of health services depending on their age and gender. For example, the average male patient requires fewer consultations than his older and infant counterparts. The table shows the weighting factors used in the standardization of workloads.

Table: Age by Sex Weights for SWPE Standardisation

Age (years)	Male	Female
less than 1	0.960	0.962
1-4	1.189	1.112
less than 10	0.688	0.699
15-24	0.633	0.938
25-44	0.729	1.012
45-64	0.963	1.199
65-74	1.355	1.623
75+	1.808	2.183

Types of Health Facility

Hospital

A hospital is an institution for healthcare typically providing specialized treatment for inpatient (or overnight) stays. Some hospitals primarily admit patients suffering from a specific disease or affection, or are reserved for the diagnosis and treatment of conditions affecting a specific age group. Others have a mandate that expands beyond offering dominantly curative and rehabilitative care services to include promotional, preventive and educational roles as part of a primary healthcare approach. Today, hospitals are usually funded by the state, health organizations (for profit or non-profit), by health insurances or by charities and by donations. Historically, however, they were often founded and funded by religious orders or charitable individuals and leaders. Hospitals are nowadays staffed by professionally trained doctors, nurses, paramedical clinicians, etc., whereas historically, this work was usually done by the founding religious orders or by volunteers.

Healthcare Center

Healthcare centres, including clinics, doctor's offices, urgent care centers and ambulatory surgery centers, serve as first point of contact with a health professional and provide outpatient medical, nursing, dental, and other types of care services.

Medical Nursing Home

Medical nursing homes, including residential treatment centers and geriatric care facilities, are health care institutions which have accommodation facilities and which engage in providing short-term or long-term medical treatment of a general or specialized nature not performed by hospitals to inpatients with any of a wide variety of medical conditions.

Pharmacies and Drug Stores

Pharmacies and drug stores comprise establishments engaged in retailing prescription or non-prescription drugs and medicines, and other types of medical and orthopaedic goods. Regulated pharmacies may be based in a hospital or clinic or they may be privately operated, and are usually staffed by pharmacists, pharmacy technicians, and pharmacy aides.

Medical Laboratory and Research

A medical laboratory or clinical laboratory is a laboratory where tests are done on biological specimens in order to get information about the health of a patient. Such laboratories may be divided into categorical departments such as microbiology, hematology, clinical biochemistry, immunology, serology, histology, cytology, cytogenetics, or virology. In many countries, there are two main types of labs that process the majority of medical specimens. Hospital laboratories are attached to a hospital, and perform tests on these patients. Private or community laboratories receive samples from general practitioners, insurance companies, and other health clinics for analysis.

A biomedical research facility is where basic research or applied research is conducted to aid the body of knowledge in the field of medicine. Medical research can be divided into two general categories: the evaluation of new treatments for both safety and efficacy in what are termed clinical trials, and all other research that contributes to the development of new treatments. The latter is termed preclinical research if its goal is specifically to elaborate knowledge for the development of new therapeutic strategies.

Hospital Ship

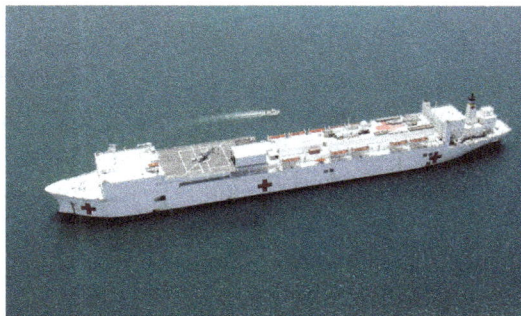

United States Navy hospital ship USNS *Comfort* in 2009.

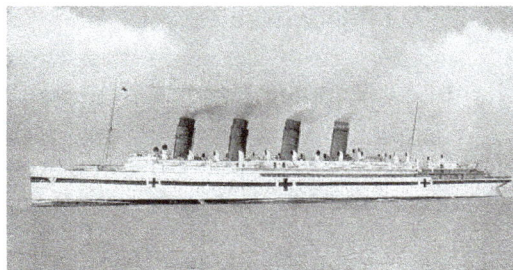

RMS *Mauretania* as hospital ship HMHS *Mauretania* during World War I.

A hospital ship is a ship designated for primary function as a floating medical treatment facility or hospital. Most are operated by the military forces (mostly navies) of various countries, as they are intended to be used in or near war zones.

Although attacking a hospital ship is a war crime, belligerent navies have the right to board such ships for inspections.

In the nineteenth century redundant warships were used as moored hospitals for seamen.

History

Early Examples

Tangier circa 1670. Hospital ships were first used during the evacuation of the port in the 1680s.

Hospital ships possibly existed in ancient times. The Athenian Navy had a ship named *Therapia*, and the Roman Navy had a ship named *Aesculapius*, their names indicating that they may have been hospital ships.

The earliest British hospital ship may have been the vessel *Goodwill*, which accompanied a Royal Navy squadron in the Mediterranean in 1608 and was used to house the sick sent aboard from other ships. However this experiment in medical care was short-lived, with *Goodwill* assigned to other tasks within a year and her complement of convalescents simply left behind at the nearest port. It was not until the mid-seventeenth century that any Royal Navy vessels were formally designated as hospital ships, and then only two throughout the fleet. These were either hired merchant ship or elderly sixth rates, with the internal bulkheads removed to create more room, and additional ports cut through the deck and hull to increase internal ventilation.

In addition to their sailing crew, these seventeenth century hospital ships were staffed by a surgeon and four surgeon's mates. The standard issue of medical supplies were bandages, soap, needles and bedpans. Patients were offered a beds or rug to rest upon, and given a clean pair of sheets. These early hospital ships were for the care of the sick rather than the wounded, with patients quartered according to their symptoms and infectious cases quarantined from the general population behind a sheet of canvas. The quality of food was very poor. In the 1690s the surgeon aboard *Siam* complained that the meat was in an advanced state of putrefaction, the biscuits were weevil-ridden and bitter, and the bread was so hard that it stripped the skin off patient's mouths.

Hospital ships were also used for the treatment of wounded soldiers fighting on land. An early example of this was during an English operation to evacuate English Tangier in 1683. An account of this evacuation was written by Samuel Pepys, an eyewitness. One of the main concerns was the evacuation of sick soldiers "and the many families and their effects to be brought off". The hospital ships *Unity* and *Welcome* sailed for England on 18 October 1683 with 114 invalid soldiers and 104 women and children, arriving at The Downs on 14 December 1683.

The number of medical personnel aboard Royal Navy hospital ships was slowly increased, with regulations issued in 1703 requiring that each vessel also carry six landsmen to act surgical assistants, and four washerwomen. A 1705 amendment provided for a further five male nurses, and requisitions from the era suggest the number of sheets per patient was increased from one to two pairs. On 8 December 1798, unfit for service as a warship, HMS *Victory* was ordered to be converted to a hospital ship to hold wounded French and Spanish prisoners of war. According to Edward Hasted in 1798, two large hospital ships (also called lazarettos), (which were the surviving hulks of forty-four gun ships) were moored in Halstow Creek in Kent. The creek is an inlet from the River Medway and the River Thames. The crew of these vessels watched over ships coming to England, which were forced to stay in the creek under quarantine to protect the country from infectious diseases including the plague.

From 1821 to 1870 the Seamen's Hospital Society provided HMS *Grampus*, HMS *Dreadnought* and HMS *Caledonia* (later renamed *Dreadnought*) as successive hospital ships moored at Deptford in London. In 1866 HMS *Hamadryad* was moored in Cardiff as a seamen's hospital, replaced in 1905 by the Royal Hamadryad Seamen's Hospital. Other redundant warships were used as hospitals for convicts and prisoners of war.

Modern Hospital Ships

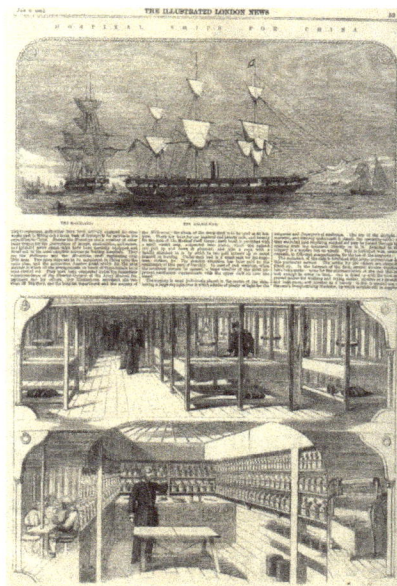

HMS *Melbourne*, the first modern hospital ship, served during the Second Opium War.
Excerpt from *The Illustrated London News* about the ship (click to read).

The institutionalization of the use of hospital ships by the Royal Navy occurred during the first half of the nineteenth century. By the standard of the medical provision available at the time for convalescent soldiers, hospital ships were generally superior in their standard of service and sanitation. It was during the Crimean War in the 1850s that the modern hospital ship began to emerge. The only military hospital available to the British forces fighting on the Crimean Peninsula was at Scutari near the Dardanelles. Over the course of the Siege of Sevastopol, almost 15,000 wounded troops were transported there from the port at Balaklava by a squadron of converted hospital ships.

The first ships to be equipped with genuine medical facilities, were the steamships HMS *Melbourne* and HMS *Mauritius*. These hospitals were manned by the Medical Staff Corps and provided services to the British expedition to China in 1860. The ships provided relatively spacious accommodation for the patients and were equipped with an operating theatre. Another early example of a hospital ship was USS *Red Rover* in the 1860s, which aided the wounded soldiers of both sides during the American Civil War.

During the Russo-Turkish War (1877–78), the British Red Cross supplied a steel-hulled ship, equipped with modern surgery equipment including chloroform and other anaesthetics and carbolic acid for antisepsis. Similar vessels accompanied the 1882 invasion of Egypt and aided American personnel during the Spanish–American War.

Hospital ships were used by both sides in the Russo-Japanese War (1904–05). It was the sighting by the Japanese of the Russian hospital ship *Orel*, correctly illuminated in accordance with regulations, that led to the decisive naval Battle of Tsushima. *Orel* was retained as a prize of war by the Japanese after the battle.

World Wars

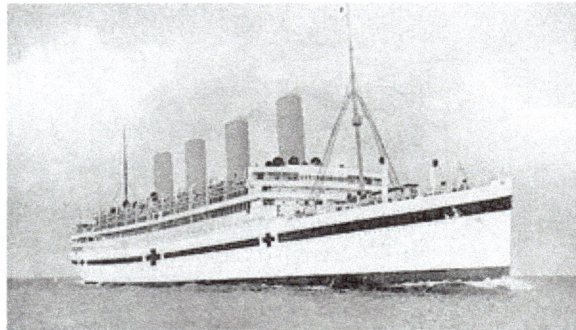

HMHS *Aquitania* in World War I service as a hospital ship.

During World War I and World War II, hospital ships were first used on a massive scale. Many passenger liners were converted for use as hospital ships. RMS *Aquitania* and HMHS *Britannic* were two famous examples of ships serving in this capacity. By the end of the First World War, The British Royal Navy had 77 such ships in service. During the Gallipoli Campaign, hospital ships were used to evacuate over 100,000 wounded personnel to Egypt.

Canada operated hospital ships in both world wars. In World War I these included SS *Letitia* (I) and HMHS *Llandovery Castle* which was deliberately sunk by a German U-boat with great loss of life, despite the hospital ship's clearly marked status. In World War II, Canada operated the hospital ship RMS *Lady Nelson* and SS *Letitia (II)*.

The first purposely built hospital ship in the U.S. Navy was USS *Relief* which was commissioned in 1921. During World War II both the United States Navy and Army operated hospital ships though with different purposes. Naval hospital ships were fully equipped hospitals designed to receive casualties direct from the battlefield and also supplied to provide logistical support to front line medical teams ashore. Army hospital ships were essentially hospital transports intended and equipped to evacuate patients from forward area Army hospitals to rear area hospitals or from those to the United States and were not equipped or staffed to handle large numbers of direct battle casualties. Three of the Navy hospital ships, USS *Comfort*, USS *Hope*, and USS *Mercy*, were less elaborately equipped than other Navy hospital ships, medically staffed by Army medical personnel and similar in purpose to the Army model.

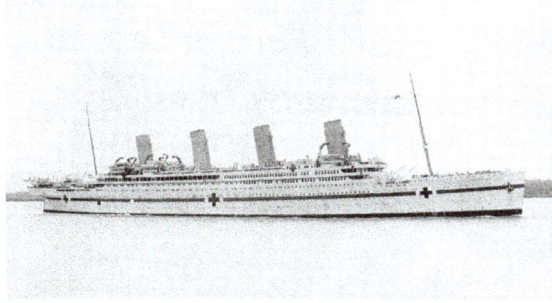

Britannic (youngest sister of *Titanic* and *Olympic*) after conversion to a hospital ship during World War I.

The last British royal yacht, the post World War II HMY *Britannia*, was ostensibly constructed in a way as to be easily convertible to a hospital ship, but this is now thought to be largely a ruse to ensure Parliamentary funding, and she never served in this role – reputedly her lifts were too small to take standard-sized stretchers.

A development of the Lun-class ekranoplan was planned for use as a mobile field hospital for rapid deployment to any ocean or coastal location at a speed of 297 knots (550 km/h). Work was 90% complete on this model, *Spasatel*, but Soviet military funding ceased and it was never completed.

Some hospital ships, such as SS *Hope* and *Esperanza del Mar*, belong to civilian agencies, and as such are not part of any navy. Mercy Ships, an international charity, do not belong to any government.

International Law

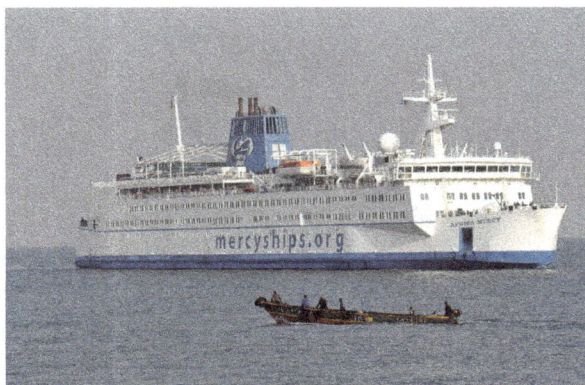

Non-government hospital ship MV *Africa Mercy*

Hospital ships were covered under the Hague Convention X of 1907. Article four of the Hague Convention X outlined the restrictions for a hospital ship:

- Ship must be clearly marked and lighted as a hospital ship

- The ship should give medical assistance to wounded personnel of all nationalities

- The ship must not be used for any military purpose

- The ship must not interfere with or hamper enemy combatant vessels

- Belligerents, as designated by the Hague Convention, can search any hospital ship to investigate violations of the above restrictions

- Belligerents will establish the location of a hospital ship

According to the San Remo Manual on International Law Applicable to Armed Conflicts at Sea, a hospital ship violating legal restrictions must be duly warned and given a reasonable time limit to comply. If a hospital ship persists in violating restrictions, a belligerent is legally entitled to capture it or take other means to enforce compliance. A non-complying hospital ship may only be fired on under the following conditions:

- Diversion or capture is not feasible

- No other method to exercise control is available

- The violations are grave enough to allow the ship to be classified as a military objective

- The damage and casualties will not be disproportionate to the military advantage.

In all other circumstances, attacking a hospital ship is a war crime.

Modern hospital ships display large Red Crosses or Red Crescents to signify their Geneva Convention protection under the laws of war. Even so, marked vessels have not been completely free from attack. Notable examples of hospital ships deliberately attacked during wartime are HMHS *Llandovery Castle* in 1915, the Soviet hospital ship *Armenia* in 1941 and AHS *Centaur* in 1943.

Current Hospital Ships

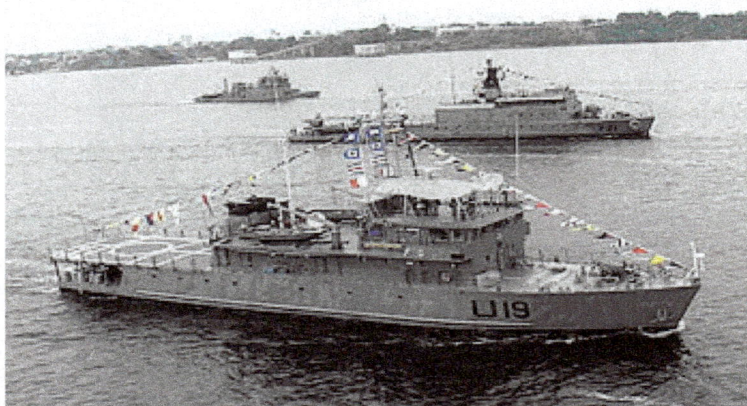

Navio de Assistência Hospitalar
Carlos Chagas

Brazilian Navy hospital ship U19 *Carlos Chagas*

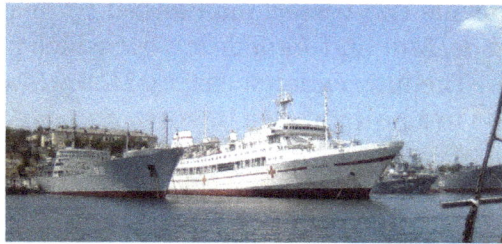
Russian Navy hospital ship *Yenisey* in Sevastopol bay

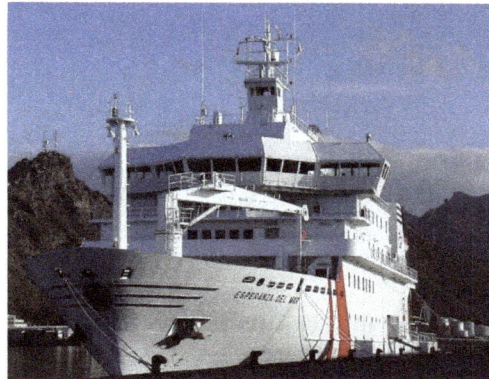

Spanish hospital ship *Esperanza Del Mar*, operated by the Ministry of Employment and Social Security.

Nation	Hospital ships
Brazil	• Six hospital ships; U15 *Pará*, U16 *Doutor Montenegro*, U18 *Oswaldo Cruz*, U19 *Carlos Chagas*, U21 *Soares de Meirelles*, U28 *Tenente Maximiano*.
China	• Two Nankang-class hospital ships: *Nankang* and *Nanyun*, being former Qiongsha-class troop transport ships modified as hospital ships in the 1980s. • *Zhuanghe* - a converted container ship capable of being fitted out for various roles. When fitted with medical facilities it is officially classed as a "medical evacuation ship". • *Daishandao*, also known as *Peace Ark* in peacetime - a converted cruise ship with 300 hospital beds, 20 intensive care units and 8 operating theatres. • Project 320 - Former Russian hospital ship *Ob* built in 1980, purchased in 2007.
Indonesia	• KRI *Dr Soeharso* - former landing ship converted to a hospital ship in 2007.
Peru	• BAP *Puno* - Former passenger and cargo ship built in 1861, converted to a hospital ship in 1976. Operates on Lake Titicaca.
Russia	• Ob' class - 3 ships *Irtysh*, *Svir* and *Yenisey* built between 1981 and 1990. Each has 7 operating rooms, 100 hospital beds and a helipad. Operated by civilian crews but with naval medical staff. Class leader *Ob* built in 1980, stricken in 1997 and sold to China in 2007.
United States	• USNS *Mercy* and USNS *Comfort*. Both operated by Military Sealift Command, their primary mission is to provide emergency on-site care for combatant forces, with a secondary mission of support for disaster relief and humanitarian operations. Each ship contains 12 operating rooms, a 1,000-bed hospital facility, digital radiological services, a medical laboratory, a pharmacy, an optometry lab, an intensive care ward, dental services, a CT scanner, a morgue, and two oxygen-producing plants. They are equipped with helicopter decks to assist with patient transport, and side ports designed to facilitate the patient transfer directly from other vessels.
Vietnam	• Hospital Ship *Khánh Hòa 01* (HQ-561) contains 20 hospital beds and has about 12 medical staff

Non-military hospital ships include two vessels maintained by Spain's Ministry of Employment and Social Security; *Esperanza del Mar* and *Juan de la Cosa* which provide medical services to the Spanish industrial fishing fleet. The international charity Mercy Ships also maintains MV *Africa Mercy*, a former ferry converted to a hospital ship in 2007.

Other Shipborne Hospitals

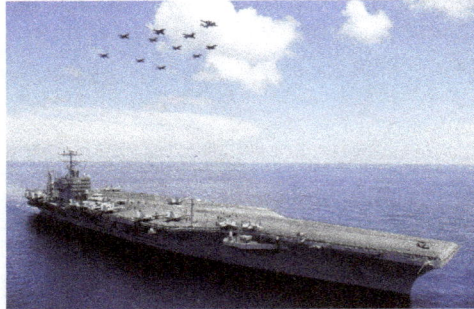

USS *Abraham Lincoln*, a *Nimitz*-class aircraft carrier

It is common for naval ships, especially large ships such as aircraft carriers and amphibious assault ships to have on-board hospitals. However, they are only one small part of the vessel's overall capability, and are used primarily for the ship's crew and its amphibious forces (and occasionally for relief missions). They do not qualify as "hospital ships", as they are not marked and designated as such, and as armed vessels they are disqualified from protection as a hospital ship under international law. Examples of these ships from various navies include;

United States Navy

Several classes of US Navy ships are equipped with on-board hospitals;

- *Nimitz*-class aircraft carrier – Each carrier has a 53-bed hospital ward, a three-bed ICU, and acts as the hospital ship for the entire carrier strike group. In one year, the medical department of USS *George Washington* handled over 15,000 out-patient visits, drew almost 27,000 labs, filled almost 10,000 prescriptions, took about 2,300 x-rays and performed 65 surgical operations. There is not much variation among the ships of the class. The first ship, USS *Nimitz* has 53 beds, plus 3 ICU beds, and the last ship, USS *George H.W. Bush* has 51 beds, plus 3 ICU beds.

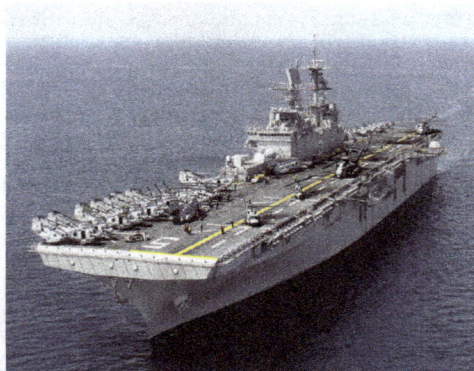

USS *Bataan*, a *Wasp*-class amphibious assault ship

- *Wasp*-class amphibious assault ship (LHD) – These ships have 6 operating rooms, 14 ICU beds, 46 hospital beds, 4 battle dressing stations, medical imaging (i.e.:X-ray), a fully functional laboratory, and a blood bank. The ship can expand its medical complement to 600 beds, making it the second largest hospital at sea, second only to actual hospital ships.

- *America*-class amphibious assault ship (LHA) – This is the newest and largest class both in the USN and the world. However, the first two ships of the class, USS *America* and USS *Tripoli*, had the size of their medical facilities reduced, in favour of larger aviation facilities. The on-board hospitals of these first two vessels will have 2 operating rooms and 24 beds. It is unknown if this design change will affect the expanded capability for additional beds, nor what size the medical facilities of future ships of the class will be.

- *San Antonio*-class amphibious transport dock (LPD) – 24 hospital beds.

- *Harpers Ferry*-class dock landing ship (LSD) – 11 hospital beds.

- *Whidbey Island*-class dock landing ship (LSD) – 8 hospital beds.

Royal Navy

- Royal Fleet Auxiliary ship RFA *Argus* – This ship would be a hospital ship were it not for its armaments. However, it is instead designated as a 'Primary Casualty Receiving Ship' (PCRS).

People's Liberation Army Navy

- Several armed Qiongsha-class cargo ships are fitted out as "ambulance transports".

- *Shichang* - a multi-role training ship built in 1997. Deck space can accommodate modular medical units and can be used as a medical treatment facility, but the primary role is aviation training. The layout is very similar to RFA *Argus*.

Dixmude, a *Mistral*-class amphibious assault ship

French Navy

- *Mistral*-class amphibious assault ship – On board hospital is NATO Echelon level-3, with 69 hospital beds, 7 ICU beds, and an additional 50 beds if needed. The ship also has medical imaging capabilities, such as X-ray, CT-scan and ultrasound.

Argentine Navy

- ARA *Almirante Irízar* - Icebreaker which can be deployed as a hospital ship.

Spanish Navy

- *Juan Carlos I* – Has a 40-bed hospital on board.

Royal Australian Navy

- *Canberra*-class landing helicopter dock – This class is based on the *Juan Carlos I*-class design, and has 2 operating rooms and a hospital ward.

Japan Maritime Self-Defense Force

- *Izumo*-class helicopter destroyer – These ships have 2 operating rooms, 2 ICU beds, 35 hospital beds, 1 battle dressing station and seval medical imaging (i.e.:X-ray) station.

- *Hyūga*-class helicopter destroyer – These ships have 1 operating room, 1 ICU bed, 8 hospital beds.

Hospital Train

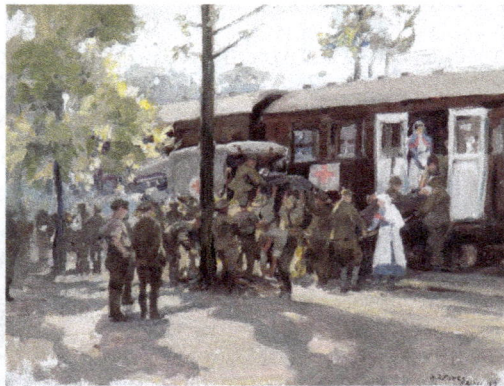

A Red Cross Train, France; wounded British soldiers are transferred from a motor ambulance to a Red Cross train, 1918, artist Harold Septimus Power.

A hospital train is a railway train with carriages equipped for the provision of healthcare. Historically this has ranged from trains equipped to transport wounded soldiers, with basic nursing and first aid facilities on board, to fully equipped mobile medical centres, sometimes including operating theatres and nursing wards.

History

Origins

The first hospital train was built during the Crimean War in the 1850s. Poorly operated logistical supply networks and inadequate health provisions for the British army encamped around the Russian port of Sevastopol caused a public outcry in England. To alleviate these problems, the Grand Crimean Central Railway was initially built by a partnership of English railway contractors led by Samuel Morton Petoin 1855, to supply ammunition and provisions to Allied soldiers. Within three weeks of the arrival of the fleet carrying materials and men the railway had started to run and in seven weeks 7 miles (11 km) of track had been completed. The railway was a major factor leading to the success of the siege. The line was surveyed by Donald Campbell.

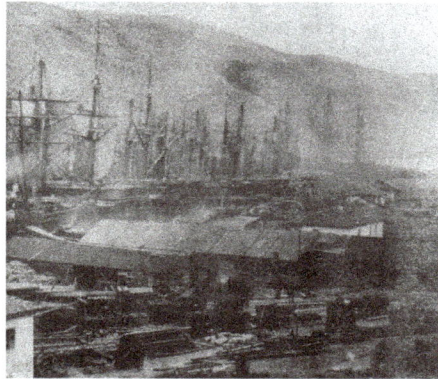

The railway yard at Balaclava, where the first hospital train operated, during the Crimean War. Photograph by Roger Fenton.

Although the railway's primary function was the supply of armaments and equipment, the train was also used for the transport of the wounded. The first such instance of this occurred on April 2, 1855, when the train was used to carry the sick and injured from the plateau down to the dock at Balaclava. Towards and during the second winter, the supplies carried by the railway were different. The siege had ended, carriage of ammunition was less important, and the supplies related more to the accommodation and comfort of the troops. These included huts to replace tents, clothing, food, books and medical supplies. Following the completion of the Sardinian branch, the railway had reached its limit. In all, it measured about 14 miles (23 km) plus a few miles of sidings and loops.

Expansion

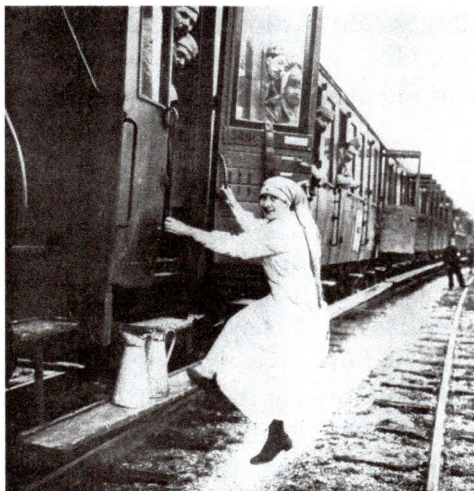

A French Red Cross train bearing sick and wounded soldiers to Paris.

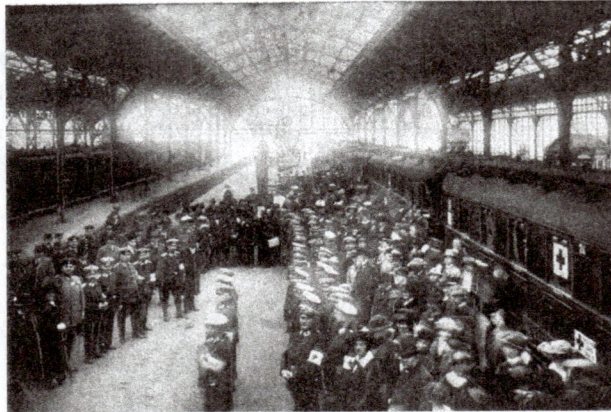

Departure of the hospital train from Lübeck on October 27, 1914

Hospital trains were subsequently used during the Franco-Austrian War, the American Civil War and the Franco-Prussian War. They were also used extensively during colonial campaigns, notably in the Anglo-Zulu War. However, these hospital trains remained primarily as troop trains, with the passengers restricted to the wounded and dying. They had little or nothing in terms of onboard medical facilities, although nurses traveled with the wounded and the carriages of the trains were painted with red crosses to indicate their humanitarian role and to prevent enemy attack.

It was during the First World War that trains began to be used as mobile medical facilities along the Western Front and other subsidiary theatres of the War. Ambulance trains were organised by the Royal Army Medical Corps with onboard surgical wards and essential medical supplies. Trains were used to evacuate over 100,000 British casualties from the battlefield at Flanders in one month of 1914 alone.

These trains were able to connect with hospital ships at French channel ports in order to repatriate wounded British soldiers back to England. There are numbers of extant journal entries from those who experienced the hospital trains of this era, many being referred to as "Great White Hospital Trains", as the carriages were often painted white or red and white.

Hospital trains were used on a large scale during the Second World War by all the major combatants and, to a more limited extent, during the Korean War. By that time, however, mobile motor transport and aerial evacuation supplanted the train as the dominant form of mobile medical provision on the battlefield.

Currently Operating Hospital Trains

The Sovereign Military Order of Malta

The Sovereign Military Order of Malta (SMOM), which is a sovereign entity (similar to an independent country, though with virtually no land), has a history of operating hospital trains through its military branch, known as the Military Corps of the Order. The operation of such trains reached its peak in the Second World War, but SMOM continues to operate such trains today. These include trains of carriages to provide shelter to refugees, with basic medical provision, and more technically equipped trains, on which a wide range of medical services may be provided.

Lifeline Express of India

The Lifeline Express is an example of a modern hospital train of a highly technologically advanced type. Operated by the Impact India Foundation since 1991, these trains have had a profound impact on Indian rural healthcare provision.

Operating in India, across the extensive network of the Indian Railways, the Lifeline trains (known colloquially as 'magic trains') move from town to town, remaining in a siding or platform at each town's railway station for perhaps a week or so, and providing advanced medical services (often beyond the capabilities of local medical centres) to those who apply for them, through a simple vetting or triage process, which ensures services are provided to those most likely to benefit. These trains include nursing wards, and full-scale operating theatres. They have resident medical and nursing staff, but for surgical procedures they rely upon the charitable provision of time and talents by Indian surgeons who spend some of their free time on board the trains for that purpose.

Chinese Eye Hospital Trains

The state-owned China Railways company currently operates four eye hospital trains, the fourth and latest being operated through the China South Locomotive and Rolling Stock Industry (Group) Corporation, and having entered service in early 2009 for the benefit of residents of the Sichuan Province. A range of ophthalmic surgeries, including the common cataract removal operation, can be provided free of charge on board the trains.

Clinic

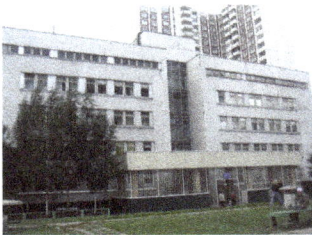

Children Polyclinic in Moscow-Novokosino.

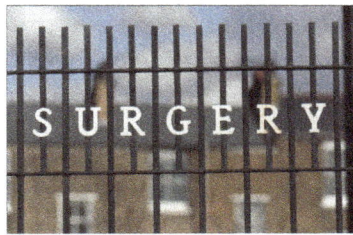

The entrance to a surgery clinic in Greenwich, London.

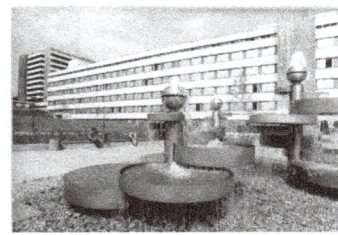

Polyclinic in Chemnitz, German Democratic Republic.

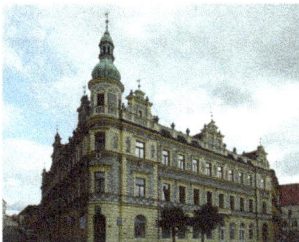

Polyclinic in Písek, Czech Republic.

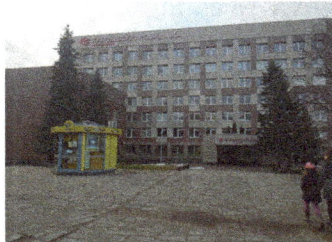

Polyclinic in Vilnius-Karoliniškės, Lithuania.

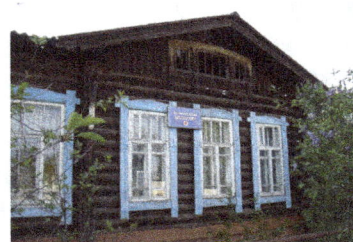

A medpunkt (health care access point) delivers primary health care to the residents of the village of Veliki Vrag in Nizhny Novgorod Oblast, Russia.

A clinic (or outpatient clinic or ambulatory care clinic) is a healthcare facility that is primarily focused on the care of outpatients. Clinics can be privately operated or publicly managed and funded. They typically cover the primary healthcare needs of populations in local communities, in contrast to larger hospitals which offer specialised treatments and admit inpatients for overnight stays.

Most commonly, the word clinic in English refers to a general medical practice, run by one or more general practitioners, but it can also mean a specialist clinic. Some clinics retain the name "clinic" even while growing into institutions as large as major hospitals or becoming associated with a hospital or medical school.

Overview

Clinics are often associated with a general medical practice run by one or several general practitioners. Other types of clinics are run by the type of specialist associated with that type: physical therapy clinics by physiotherapists and psychology clinics by clinical psychologists, and so on for each health profession. (This can even hold true for certain services outside the medical field: for example, legal clinics are run by lawyers.)

Some clinics are operated in-house by employers, government organizations, or hospitals, and some clinical services are outsourced to private corporations which specialize in providing health services. In China, for example, owners of such clinics do not have formal medical education. There were 659,596 village clinics in China in 2011.

Health care in India, China, Russia and Africa is provided to those countries' vast rural areas by mobile health clinics or roadside dispensaries, some of which integrate traditional medicine. In India these traditional clinics provide ayurvedic medicine and unani herbal medical practice. In each of these countries, traditional medicine tends to be a hereditary practice.

The word *clinic* derives from Ancient Greek *klinein* meaning to slope, lean or recline. Hence *klinē* is a couch or bed and *klinikos* is a physician who visits his patients in their beds. In Latin, this became *clīnicus*.

An early use of the word clinic was "one who receives baptism on a sick bed".

Function

The function of clinics differs from country to country. For instance, a local general practice run by a single general practitioner provides primary health care and is usually run as a for-profit business by the owner, whereas a government-run specialist clinic may provide subsidised or specialised health care.

Some clinics function as a place for people with injuries or illnesses to come and be seen by a triage nurse or other health worker. In these clinics, the injury or illness may not be serious enough to require a visit to an emergency room (ER), but the person can be transferred to one if needed.

Treatment at these clinics is often less expensive than it would be at a casualty department. Also, unlike an ER these clinics are often not open on a 24 x 7 x 365 basis. They sometimes have access to diagnostic equipment such as X-ray machines, especially if the clinic is part of a larger facility. Doctors at such clinics can often refer patients to specialists if the need arises.

Large Outpatient Clinics

Large outpatient clinics vary in size, but can be as large as hospitals.

Function

Typical large outpatient clinics house general medical practitioners (GPs) such as doctors and nurses to provide ambulatory care and some acute care services but lack the major surgical and pre- and post-operative care facilities commonly associated with hospitals.

Besides GPs, if a clinic is a polyclinic, it can house outpatient departments of some medical specialties, such as gynecology, dermatology, ophthalmology, otolaryngology, neurology, pulmonology, cardiology, and endocrinology. In some university cities, polyclinics contain outpatient departments for the entire teaching hospital in one building.

Internationally

Large outpatient clinics are a common type of healthcare facility in many countries, including France, Germany (long tradition), Switzerland, and most of the countries of Central and Eastern Europe (often using a mixed Soviet-German model), as well as in former Soviet republics such as Russia and Ukraine; and in many countries across Asia and Africa.

Recent Russian governments have attempted to replace the polyclinic model introduced during Soviet times with a more western model. However, this has failed.

India has also set up huge numbers of polyclinics for former defence personnel. The network envisages 426 polyclinics in 343 districts of the country which will benefit about 33 lakh (3.3 million) ex-servicemen residing in remote and far-flung areas.

Polyclinics are also the backbone of Cuba's primary care system and have been credited with a role in improving that nation's health indicators.

Types

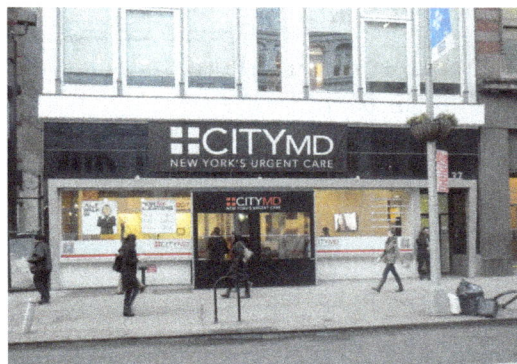

Storefront clinic in Manhattan.

There are many different types of clinics providing outpatient services. Such clinics may be public (government-funded) or private medical practices.

- A CLSC are in Quebec; they are a type of free clinic funded by the provincial government; they provide service not covered by Canada's healthcare plan including social workers

- In the United States, a free clinic provides free or low-cost healthcare for those without insurance.

- A retail-based clinic is housed in supermarkets and similar retail outlets providing walk-in health care, which may be staffed by nurse practitioners.

- A general out-patient clinic offers general diagnoses or treatments without an overnight stay.

- A polyclinic provides a range of healthcare services (including diagnostics) without need of an overnight stay

- A specialist clinic provides advanced diagnostic or treatment services for specific diseases or parts of the body. This type contrasts with general out-patient clinics.

  o A sexual health clinic deals with sexual health related problems, such as prevention and treatment of sexually transmitted infections.

  o A fertility clinic aims to help women and couples to become pregnant.

  o An abortion clinic is a medical facility providing abortion and related medical services to women.

  o An ambulatory surgery clinic offers outpatient or same day surgery services, usually for surgical procedures less complicated than those requiring hospitalization.

Examples

- Tavistock Clinic, part of the British NHS, was founded in the 1920s. One of its most celebrated members was R D Laing.

- The Suitcase Clinic, the Berkeley Free Clinic, and the Haight Ashbury Free Clinic are examples of free clinics.

- Christian Medical College & Hospital in Vellore, India has extensive roadside dispensaries and began as a one-bed clinic in 1900.

- The Edmonton Clinic is a joint venture of the University of Alberta and government health care body Capital health, expected to be completed in 2011.

- The Shyness Clinic founded by Zimbardo to assist those disabled by public or private shyness.

- La Borde clinic in the Loire valley France, is an innovative psychiatric clinic where patients are liberated to actively participate in the running of the facility.

- The Mayo Clinic, Cleveland Clinic, Marshfield Clinic and Lahey Clinic are examples of comprehensive health care systems, all having begun as much smaller group practices that have since grown into large medical programs in the United States, whilst retaining their names.

- The Gary Burnstein Community Health Clinic, a non-profit, volunteer-supported Free Clinic in Pontiac, Michigan.

- The Balaji Physiotherapy & Rehabilitation Clinic "for muscle, joint, back pain, stroke and spine rehabilitation treatments" in Jodhpur, Rajasthan, India.

Free Clinic

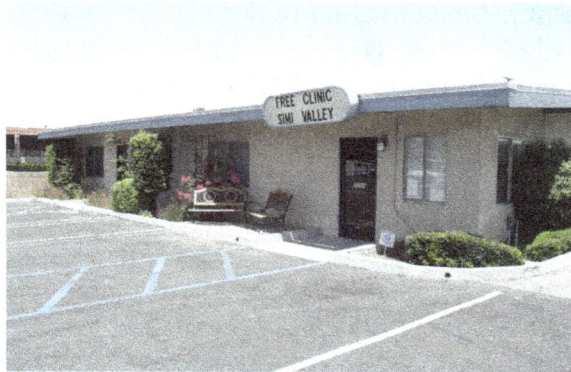

Free Clinic of Simi Valley, Simi Valley, California

A free clinic is a health care facility in the United States offering services to economically disadvantaged individuals for free or at a nominal cost. Core staff members may hold full-time paid positions, however, most of the staff a patient will encounter are volunteers drawn from the local medical community. Care is provided free of cost to persons who have limited incomes, no health insurance and do not qualify for Medicaid or Medicare. To offset costs, some clinics charge a nominal fee to those whose income is deemed sufficient to pay a fee. Many free clinics offer services to underinsured individuals; meaning those who have only limited medical coverage (such as catastrophic care coverage, but not regular coverage), or who have insurance, but their policies include high medical deductibles that they are unable to afford. Clinics often use the term "underinsured" to describe the working poor.

Most free clinics provide treatment for routine illness or injuries; and long-term chronic conditions such as high blood pressure, diabetes, asthma and high cholesterol. Many also provide a limited range of medical testing, prescription drug assistance, women's health care, and dental care. Free clinics do not function as emergency care providers, and most do not handle employment related injuries. Few if any free clinics offer care for chronic pain as that would require them to dispense narcotics. For a free clinic such care is almost always cost-prohibitive. Handling narcotics requires a high level of physical security for the staff and building along with more paperwork and government regulation compared to what other prescription medications require.

History

The modern notion of a free clinic began in the 1960s in San Francisco when Dr. David Smith founded the Haight Ashbury Free Clinics in 1967 during the summer of love in the Haight Ashbury district. Free clinics quickly spread to other California cities and the rest of the United States. In 1972 a meeting was held in Washington DC where clinic staff from around the country gathered and listened to speakers including Dr. Smith. At this meeting the slogan "Health Care is a Right Not a Privilege" emerged as a theme.

During the 1970s and 80s free clinics continued to evolve and change to meet the needs of their individual communities, however some were unable to survive. Each free clinic was unique in its development and services, based on the particular needs and resources of the local community. There is a saying among free clinic organizations that, if you have been to one free clinic, you have been to all free clinics. The common denominator is that care is made possible through the service of volunteers, the donation of goods and community support. Funding is generally donated on the local level and there is little —if any— government funding. Some free clinics were established to provide medical services in the inner cities while others opened in the suburbs and many student-run free clinics have emerged that serve the under-served as well as provide a medical training site for students in the health professions.

In 2001 the National Association of Free and Charitable Clinics (NAFC) was founded in Washington, D.C. to advocate for the issues and concerns of free and charitable clinics. Free clinics are defined by the NAFC as "safety-net health care organizations that utilize a volunteer/staff model to provide a range of medical, dental, pharmacy, vision and/or behavioral health services to economically disadvantaged individuals. Such clinics are 501(c)3 tax-exempt organizations, or operate as a program component or affiliate of a 501(c)(3) organization." In time various state and regional organizations where formed including the Free Clinics of the Great Lakes Region, Lone Star Association of Charitable Clinic (Texas), North Carolina Association of Free Clinics, Ohio Association of Free Clinics and the Virginia Association of Free Clinics. In 2005 Empowering Community Healthcare Outreach (ECHO) was established to assist churches and other community organizations start and run free and charitable clinics.

Health Care Safety Net

Some free clinics specialize in providing primary care (acute care), while others focus on long-term chronic health issues, and many do both. Most free clinics start out seeing patients only one or two days per week, and then expand as they find additional volunteers. Because they rely on volunteers, most are only open a few hours per day; primarily in the late afternoon and early evening. Many free clinics are faith-based, meaning they are sponsored by and affiliated with a specific church or religious denomination, or they are interfaith and draw support from several different denominations or religions.

Free clinics rely on donations for financial support. The amount of money they take in through donations to a large degree determines how many patients they are able to see. Because they are unlikely to have the resources to see everyone who might need their help, they usually limit who they are willing to see to just those from their own community and the surrounding areas, and especially in chronic care will only see patients from within a limited set of medical conditions. For example, they will see a patient for diabetes, but are not in a position to help with cancer. Some will see only patents that have no insurance, while others will see the underinsured as well.

Free clinics function as health care safety nets, meaning they provide essential services regardless of the patient's ability to pay. Hospital emergency rooms are required by federal law to treat everyone regardless of their ability to pay, so people who lack the means to pay for care often seek treatment in emergency rooms for minor ailments. Treating people in the ER is expensive and it ties up resources designed for emergencies. When a community has a free clinic, hospitals can steer patients to the clinic who otherwise would have been seen in the ER, patients who have a simple ear ache, pink eye, strep throat, flu, etc. For this reason most hospitals are supportive of free clinics. Hospitals are a primary source for equipment and supplies for free clinics. When they upgrade equipment, they will often donate the older equipment to the local free clinic. In addition some hospitals supply most or all of a local clinics day-to-day medical supplies, and some do lab work free of cost as well.

Location

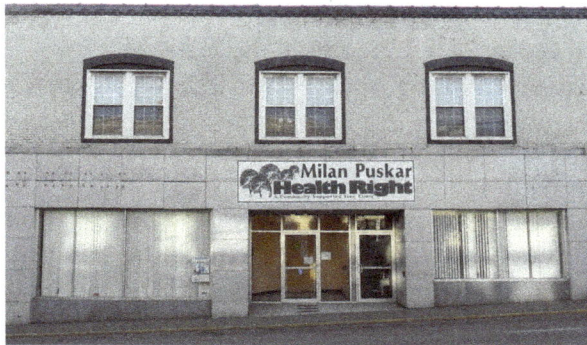

Milan Puskar Health Right free clinic in Morgantown, West Virginia

Free clinics are usually located near the people they are trying to serve. In most cases they are located near other nonprofits that serve the same target community such as food-banks, Head Start, Goodwill Industries, the Salvation Army and public housing. Because free clinics often refer people to other medical facilities for lab work, dentistry, and other services, they are usually found in the same area of town as those medical facilities. Almost all free clinics have working agreements with the other facilities that are willing to assist with the clinics mission. Being close to the other medical facilities makes it easier for patients to get from one to the other. Being close to other medical facilities also makes it easier to find medically trained volunteers.

Most free clinics start out using donated space; others start by renting or leasing space. In time and with enough community support, many go on to acquire their own buildings. Donated space may be an entire building, or it might be a couple of rooms within a church, hospital, or another business. Because the clinic will house confidential medical records, prescription medications, and must remain as clean as possible, donated space is usually set aside for the sole use of the clinic even when the clinic is closed.

Medical Malpractice Liability

Free clinics can be granted medical malpractice coverage through the Federal Tort Claims Act (FTCA). FTCA coverage includes health care professionals who are acting as volunteers. In addition it covers officers, board members, clinic employees, and individual contractors. Medical malpractice coverage does not occur automatically, each organization must be "deemed" eligible by the US Department of Health and Human Services. To be eligible the clinic must be an IRS recognized nonprofit, that does not accept payments from insurance companies, the government, or other organizations for the services it performs. It also must not charge patients for services. It may receive donations from anyone and any organization; the stipulation is that it may not receive financial reimbursement for service rendered, which by definition a free clinic does not.

The Volunteer Protection Act of 1997 provides immunity from tort claims such as negligence, bodily injury, pain and suffering that might be filed against the volunteers of nonprofit organizations. Thus, volunteers working on behalf of a nonprofit free clinic are covered under the Volunteer Protection Act from most liability claims.

Individual states may offer additional legal protections to free clinics, usually under the states Good Samaritan laws. Free clinics must still carry general liability insurance, to cover non-medical liability, such as slips and falls in the parking lot.

Prescription Assistance Programs

Some pharmaceutical companies offer assistance programs for the drugs they manufacture. These programs allow those who are unable to pay for their medications to receive prescription drugs for free or at a greatly reduced cost. Many free clinics work to qualify patients on behalf of these programs. In some cases the clinic receive and then distribute the medications themselves, in others they verify that the patient is eligible for the program, and the medication is then shipped to the patient, or patient receives the medication from a local pharmacy.

Some free clinics sole mission is to help those who do not have prescription drug coverage, and cannot afford for their medications, to enroll in prescription assistance programs. Such clinics are known as "clinics without walls" because they dispense with the need to have their own building, exam rooms, or clinical equipment.

Dentistry

Some free clinics are able to assist with dental problems. This is handled either at the clinic itself, if the clinic has its own dental facilities and a dentist; or it is facilitated through a partnership with one or more local dentist who are willing to take referred patients for free. For example, a clinic might have ten local dentists who will each accept two patients per month, so this allows the clinic to treat a total of twenty dental patients each month.

Some clinics use a referral system to handle other forms of specialized medical care.

Student-run Clinics

There is an academic model for free clinics. The Society of Student-Run Free Clinics (SSRFC) hosts a national inter-professional platform for student-run clinics. This allows the sharing of ideas, collaborate on research, information about funding resources and encourages the expansion of existing clinics as well as the cultivate of the new ones. The SSRFC faculty network works to facilitate collaboration between student-run free clinics.

Nurse-led Clinic

A nurse-led clinic is any outpatient clinic that is run or managed by registered nurses, usually nurse practitioners or Clinical Nurse Specialists in the UK. Nurse-led clinics have assumed distinct roles over the years, and examples exist within hospital outpatient departments, public health clinics and independent practice environments.

Definition

A broad definition of a nurse-led clinic defines these clinics based on what nursing activities are performed at the site. Nurses within a nurse-led clinic assume their own patient case-loads, provide an educative role to patients to promote health, provide psychological support, monitor the patient's condition and perform nursing interventions. Advanced practice registered nurses, usually nurse practitioners, may have expanded roles within these clinics, depending on the scope of practice defined by their state, provincial or territorial government.

Overview

The recent growth of nurse-led clinics is considered an emerging area of nursing practice; they were originally discussed in nursing journals in the 1980s, and developed over the 1990s into practice areas that have generated financial, legal and professional challenges over the years. There has been recent growth of nurse-led clinics both within hospitals and in the community. However, that growth has been unequal across different legislative regions. As an example, Canada's only known nurse-led clinics exist in Ontario. Unlike many clinics which exist in the United States, Ontario's clinics have been met with some criticism from the Ontario Medical Association and some family physicians who view nurse-led clinics to be unproven innovations in primary care.

In the UK, advanced nursing practice developed in the 1980s in response to increased health needs and cost, and in keeping with health policy. A later impetus came from the "New deal for junior doctors" which was a government response to the European Community directive to reduce junior doctors' hours of work.

Nurse-led clinics typically focus on chronic disease management: conditions where regular follow-up and expertise is required, but also where a patient may not necessarily need to see a physician at every visit. Most nurse-led clinics use nursing theory and knowledge to educate patients and form care plans to manage their conditions.

Review of Evidence

Nurse-led clinics have a brief history of evaluation in scientific literature. Not only is there a large amount of heterogeneity between nurse-led clinics, but there are also different educational backgrounds for nurses who wish to enter these roles.

In a partially blind randomized controlled trial, adult patients with Type II Diabetes were found to have better control of hypertension and hyperlipidemia in a nurse-led clinic when compared to conventional follow-up care. A related study also found that nurse-led clinics were more effective than conventional care in controlling hypertension for adult patients with Type II Diabetes and uncontrolled hypertension. Generally, it was found that most patients experienced improved outcomes following nurse-led clinic consultation, with the best improvement rates found for wound care and continence clinics.

Many nurse-led clinics have also been associated with enhanced patient satisfaction with care. A nurse-led clinic for intractable constipation in pediatric populations was compared to a pediatric gastroenterology clinic, illustrating that parent satisfaction was significantly higher for those who attended the nurse-led clinic. This has also been shown in rheumatology nurse-led clinics

In areas where nursing practice may require additional support to maintain patient safety, some nurse-led clinics have implemented decision support tools, computerized systems and evidence-based algorithms to support their practice. Nurse-led clinics which utilize computerized decision support tools to manage oral anticoagulation dosages were found be to as effective as hospital-based clinics for INR control and stability.

In the UK, nurse-led care has been established in many chronic conditions such as diabetes, COPD and musculoskletal disorders. Treatment guidelines in rheumatoid arthritis for example, specify the role of the nurse in managing the disease.

The evidence for the effectiveness of nurse-led intervention is growing and increasingly supported by randomised controlled trials and systematic reviews.

Walk-in Clinic

A walk-in clinic describes a very broad category of medical facilities only loosely defined as those that accept patients on a walk-in basis and with no appointment required. A number of healthcare service providers fall under the walk-in clinic umbrella including urgent care centers, retail clinics and even many free clinics or community health clinics. Walk-in clinics offer the advantages of being accessible and often inexpensive. However amongst the negative aspects are that walk-in clinics provide poor quality healthcare as opposed to professional healthcare such as regular doctors and hospitals. Other disadvantages may include the urgency to make the patient's visit as quick as possible in order to reduce the long waiting list of walk-ins at the clinic, which may fail to fulfill the purpose of the visit.

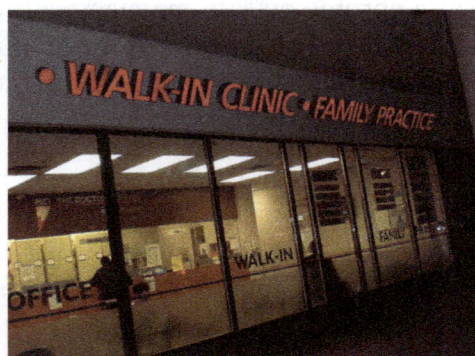

A walk-in clinic in Toronto, Canada.

It is estimated that there are nearly 11,000 walk-in clinics in America, although it is impossible to calculate an exact number given the variable and ill-defined nature of the category. Urgent care centers make up the largest percentage of walk-in clinics in America with an estimated 9,000 locations nationwide.

In fact, consumers often erroneously refer to all walk-in clinics as urgent care centers, and vice versa. Retail clinics are the next most prevalent in the industry with 1,443 locations as of July 1, 2013.

Services

Urgent care clinics are usually led by physicians. The much smaller category of retail clinics, which are stand-alone clinics located inside large retail stores or shopping malls, tend to be headed by nurse practitioners. The significantly higher price for an urgent care visit compared to a retail clinic visit is largely attributed to this difference in staffing.

All types of walk-in clinics provide basic medical services, such as routine vaccinations, evaluation of cold and flu symptoms, and treatment for less severe physical injuries. Urgent care centers normally provide more services, such as X-ray testing for suspected pneumonia or broken bones.

Access to the patient's regular medical records depends on the agreements that the clinic has with other organizations. For example, a walk-in clinic that is part of or affiliated with a hospital or larger clinic may have full access to all the medical records belonging to the larger institution, while an independent walk-in clinic may not have access any patient records except those related to previous visits to that walk-in clinic. This lack of access can prevent healthcare providers from recognizing chronic problems.

Major Companies

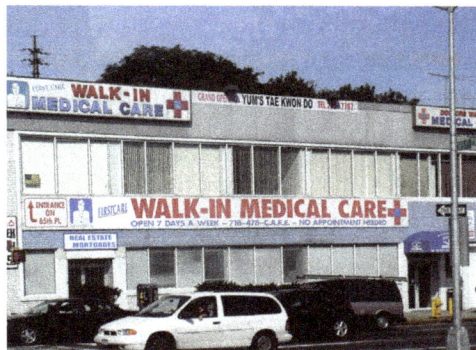

Walk-in Medical Care Center in New York City, Queens Boulevard

According to Merchant Medicine's U.S. Walk-in Clinic Market Report for July 2013, the following are the top twenty walk-in clinic brands:

Company Brand	# of Clinics
MinuteClinic (CVS)	665
Healthcare Clinic at Walgreens	371
Concentra	309
US Healthworks	145
AFC Doctors Express	140
MedExpress	112
The Little Clinic	93

Company Brand	# of Clinics
NextCare	87
Target Clinic	54
FastMed	53
Doctors Care	52
Patient First	46
CareSpot	45
RediClinic	30
Physicians Immediate Care	29
Hometown	27
FastCare	25
Baptist Express Care at Walmart	18
WellNow	17
DR Walk-In Medical Clinics	13

Controversies

The existence of walk-in clinics has been controversial. Doctors acknowledge that Minute Clinics and other retail-based clinics are convenient. They admit that the clinics are cutting into their own income. However, doctors say they are trying to build a relationship with their patients, meet them regularly, and follow up on problems. The clinics interfere with that relationship and fragment health care. Furthermore, said pediatrician Claire McCarthy, "Sometimes a minor thing isn't so minor." The clinics don't have the patient's medical record, and don't know the history. A swollen knee, if it is part of a pattern, might be a sign of arthritis. The American Academy of Pediatrics has recommended that parents do not use retail-based clinics for their children

Urgent Care

Urgent care is a category of walk-in clinic focused on the delivery of ambulatory care in a dedicated medical facility outside of a traditional emergency room. Urgent care centers primarily treat injuries or illnesses requiring immediate care, but not serious enough to require an ER visit. Urgent care centers are distinguished from similar ambulatory healthcare centers such as emergency departments and convenient care clinics by their scope of conditions treated and available facilities on-site. While urgent care centers are usually not open 24-hours a day, 70% of centers in the United States open by 8:00 am or earlier and 95% close after 7:00 pm.

History of Urgent Care in the United States

The initial urgent care centers opened in the 1970s. Since then, this healthcare industry sector rapidly expanded to approximately 10,000 centers. Many centers were started by emergency medicine physicians, responding to a public need for convenient access to unscheduled medical care. A significant factor for the increase of these centers is significant monetary savings when compared to ERs. Many managed care organizations (MCOs) now encourage or even require customers to utilize urgent care options. As of 2014, the urgent care industry is worth an estimated $14.5 Billion.

Demographic Features of Urgent Care Patients and Providers

In 2014, US communities with non-hospital-based urgent care centers (UCCs) were mainly urban, located in areas with higher income levels and higher levels of private insurance. Kaissi et al considered local multi-hospital systems in Florida, Maryland, Nevada, Texas, Virginia and Washington. In 2012 50% of 117 hospital-based "clusters" included either UCCs, retail clinics, or both. 57% of systems in Washington operated an UCC, compared to 36% of systems in Washington, while systems in Florida had the largest share of UCCs (17.6%). Authors noted unexplained state-by-state variation in hospital system partnership with UCC and retail clinic models. Corwin et al considered Medicare beneficiaries presenting to an UCC (n=1,426,354) emergency department (ED) (n=334,841) or physicians office (n=8,359,498) with upper respiratory or urinary tract infections, bronchitis, sprains or contusions, and back or arthritic pain, in 2012. Patients who presented to an ED were more likely to be female (67% of ED presentations) compared to those who presented to a UCC or physicians office (65% and 64% respectively). Patients who presented to an UCC were significantly more likely to be aged over 85 (27%, compared to 15% of physicians office presentations, and 13% of ED presentations) or Black (11%, compared to 6% of physicians office presentations, and 4% of ED presentations). In 2014, 3.1% of Family Physicians in the United States worked primarily in UCCs, with a male:female ratio of workforce is 6:7, and an urban:rural ratio of 2:1. This compares to 3.6% of Family Physicians working primarily in Emergency Care, with a male:female ratio of 5:3 and urban:rural ratio approaching 1:2.

Criteria for Urgent Care Centers

Both the Urgent Care Association of America (UCAOA) and the American Academy of Urgent Care Medicine (AAUCM) have established criteria for urgent care centers and the physicians that operate them. Each share similar qualifying criteria including:

- Must accept walk-in patients during business hours

- Treat a broad spectrum of illnesses and injuries, as well as perform minor medical procedures

- Have a licensed physician operating as the medical director

- Be open 7 days a week

- Have on-site diagnostic equipment, including phlebotomy and x-ray

- Contain multiple exam rooms

- Various ethical and business standards

The UCAOA program is called Urgent Care Certification and the AAUCM is called Urgent Care Center Accreditation.

Organized Medicine and Urgent Care

The Urgent Care Association of America (UCAOA) holds an annual spring convention and an annual fall conference. Many leaders of organized urgent care anticipate the establishment of urgent care as a fully recognized specialty.

Urgent Care Management Monthly hosts a bi-annual conference, teaching doctors, investors, and owners about the business side of an urgent care center. Urgent Care Management Monthly (UCMM) is the official publication for urgent care management, with discussions on topics such as billing, staffing, marketing, accounting, and logistics.

JUCM, The Journal of Urgent Care Medicine is the Official Publication of the Urgent Care Association of America (UCAOA). Each issue contains peer-reviewed clinical and practice management articles.

Board of Certification in Urgent Care Medicine (BCUCM) provides board certification for physicians with requisite training and experience. Urgent Care College of Physicians (UCCOP)

Postgraduate Training

In 2006, the Urgent Care Association of America sponsored the first fellowship training program in urgent care medicine. A collaboration between the Department of Family Medicine University Hospitals of Cleveland / Case School of Medicine, the Urgent Care Association of America (UCAOA), and University Primary and Specialty Care Practices, Inc. in Cleveland, Ohio made this fellowship possible. The program was partially funded by an unrestricted grant from the Urgent Care Association of America. Fellowship physicians receive training in many disciplines, including: adult emergencies, pediatric emergencies, wound & injury evaluation and treatment, occupational medicine, urgent care procedures, and care center business aspects. In 2007, the Urgent Care Association of America (UCAOA) sponsored a second fellowship opportunity through the University of Illinois. The one-year fellowships are open to graduates of accredited Family Medicine and Med/Peds residencies.

Staffing and Services

Unlike other walk-in clinics such as retail clinics, urgent care centers are generally staffed by a physician and supported by nurses, physician assistants and medical assistants. Sixty-five percent of urgent care centers have at least one physician on-site at all times.

Of the physicians that staff urgent care centers, 47.8% are family medicine, 30.1% are emergency medicine and 7.6% are internal medicine.

With these licensed physician on-site, urgent care centers are able to offer a wide range of services including broken bones, moderate cuts and lacerations requiring stitches, and most common injuries and illnesses. These services, of course, are made possible with the diagnostic equipment and x-ray machines typically found at an urgent care.

Of course, the urgent care centers are not an emergency room. They do not offer surgical services, as a rule- particularly invasive surgical procedures (more than cutaneous or subcutaneous procedures- those involving body organs and organ parts, and/or deep penetration of deep fascia, tendons, ligaments, bursae, joints, muscles, or bones), any procedures requiring the use of regional or general anesthesia (more than topical local anesthesia), those procedures requiring a full operating room or suite, having lengthy recovery times, or requiring more than the level of imaging or specialists available at the center.

That said, an estimated 13.7 to 27.1 percent of all emergency department visits could take place at an urgent care center or a retail clinic, generating a potential cost savings of approximately $4.4 billion annually, according to a 2010 study in Health Affairs.

Ownership

The majority of urgent care centers are owned by physicians or physician groups, however, more corporations and investment banks are acquiring urgent care centers and creating regional and national brands in the industry. The following is a breakdown of urgent care ownership following a 2012 study by the UCAOA:

- 35.4 percent of centers owned by physicians or physician groups, down from 50 percent in 2010

- 30.5 percent owned by a corporation, up from 13.5 percent in 2010

- 25.2 percent owned by a hospital

- 4.4 percent owned by a non-physician individual

- 2.2 percent owned by a franchise

Codes for Urgent Care

In recent years the American Medical Association approved the code UCM (Urgent Care Medicine). This code allows physicians to self-designate as specializing in urgent care medicine. Services rendered in an urgent care center may be designated, using the place of service code -20 (POS -20) on the CMS-1500 form, as submitted to third-party payers. The Centers for Medicare & Medicaid Services (CMS) have designated two specific codes to apply to urgent care centers: S9083 (global fee for urgent care centers) and S9088 (services rendered in an urgent care center).

Inpatient Care

Inpatient care is the care of patients whose condition requires admission to a hospital. Progress in modern medicine and the advent of comprehensive out-patient clinics ensure that patients are only admitted to a hospital when they are extremely ill or have severe physical trauma.

Progress

Patients enter inpatient care mainly from previous ambulatory care such as referral from a family doctor, or through emergency medicine departments. The patient formally becomes an "inpatient" at the writing of an admission note.

Likewise, it is formally ended by writing a discharge note.

Planning for Patient Discharge

Healthcare professionals involved in rehabilitation are often involved in discharge planning for patients. When considering patient discharge, there are a number of factors to take into consideration: the patient's current state, their place of residence and the type of support available. When considering the patient's current state, although the patient may be eligible for discharge it is important to examine factors such as the likelihood of re-injury to avoid higher health care costs. Patients' homes should also be visited and examined before they are discharged from the hospital to determine any immediate challenges and corresponding goals, adaptations and assistive devices that need to be implemented. Follow-up appointments should also be coordinated with the patient prior to discharge to monitor the patient's progress as well as any potential complications that may have arisen.

History

Inpatient care goes back to 230 BC in India where Ashoka founded 18 hospitals. The Romans also adopted the concept of inpatient care by building a specialized temple for sick patients in 291 AD on the island of Tiber.

It is believed the first inpatient care in North America was provided by the Spanish in the Dominican Republic in 1502; the Hospital de Jesús Nazareno in Mexico City was founded in 1524 and is still providing inpatient care.

Perhaps the most famous provider of inpatient care was Florence Nightingale who was the leading advocate for improving medical care in the mid-19th century.

Ms. Nightingale received notoriety during the Crimean War where she and 38 women volunteer nurses traveled to Crimea to treat wounded soldiers. During her first winter at the hospital 4077 soldiers died in the hospital there. She would use this experience to change the course of inpatient care by focusing on improving sanitary conditions and better living conditions within the hospital.

Florence Nightingale became known as "The Lady with the Lamp" and is still considered the founder of modern nursing. The Nightingale School of Nursing continues today and her image is the one depicted each year on nurses' day.

Hospitalist Medicine

The original model for inpatient care required a family physician to admit a patient and then make rounds and manage the patient's care during their hospital stay. That model is rapidly being replaced by hospitalist medicine a term first used by Dr. Robert Wachter in an article written for the New England Journal of Medicine in 1996.

The concept of hospitalist medicine provides around the clock inpatient care from physicians whose sole practice is the hospital itself. They work with the community of primary care physicians to provide inpatient care and transition patients back to the care of their primary care provider upon discharge. Using this approach, primary care physicians are no longer required to make rounds or be on call.

Today, hospitalist medicine is the fastest growing segment of medicine and is being adopted by hospitals worldwide for inpatient care.

Statistics

In 2011, there were approximately 39 million inpatient stays in the United States, with a national aggregate cost of $387 billion. U.S. programs Medicare and Medicaid bore responsibility for 63 percent of these total aggregate costs.

In 2011, approximately one quarter of hospital stays in the United States were in the intensive care unit; these accounted for nearly half the aggregate total hospital charges that year.

Medical Home

American College of Physicians

The medical home, also known as the patient-centered medical home (PCMH), is a team-based health care delivery model led by a health care provider that is intended to provide comprehensive and continuous medical care to patients with the goal of obtaining maximized health outcomes. It is described in the "Joint Principles" as "an approach to providing comprehensive primary care for children, youth and adults."

The provision of medical homes is intended to allow better access to health care, increase satisfaction with care, and improve health.

The "Joint Principles" that popularly define a PCMH were established through the efforts of the American Academy of Pediatrics (AAP), American Academy of Family Physicians (AAFP), American College of Physicians (ACP), and American Osteopathic Association (AOA) in 2007. Care coordination is an essential component of the PCMH. Care coordination requires additional resources such as health information technology and appropriately-trained staff to provide coordinated care through team-based models. Additionally, payment models that compensate PCMHs for their functions devoted to care coordination activities and patient-centered care management that fall outside the face-to-face patient encounter may help encourage further coordination.

History

The concept of the "medical home" has evolved since the first introduction of the term by the American Academy of Pediatrics in 1967. At the time, it was envisioned as a central source for all the medical information about a child, especially those with special needs. Efforts by Calvin C.J. Sia, MD, a Honolulu-based pediatrician, in pursuit of new approaches to improve early childhood development in Hawaii in the 1980s laid the groundwork for an Academy policy statement in 1992 that defined a medical home largely the way Sia conceived it: a strategy for delivering the family-centered, comprehensive, continuous, and coordinated care that all infants and children deserve. In 2002, the organization expanded and operationalized the definition.

In 2002, seven U.S. national family medicine organizations created the *Future of Family Medicine* project to "transform and renew the specialty of family medicine." Among the recommendations of the project was that every American should have a "personal medical home" through which they could receive acute, chronic, and preventive health services. These services should be "accessible, accountable, comprehensive, integrated, patient-centered, safe, scientifically valid, and satisfying to both patients and their physicians."

As of 2004, one study estimated that if the *Future of Family Medicine* recommendations were followed (including implementation of personal medical homes), "health care costs would likely decrease by 5.6 percent, resulting in national savings of 67 billion dollars per year, with an improvement in the quality of the health care provided." A review of this assertion, published later the same year, determined that medical homes are "associated with better health,... with lower overall costs of care and with reductions in disparities in health."

By 2005, the American College of Physicians had developed an "advanced medical home" model. This model involved the use of evidence-based medicine, clinical decision support tools, the Chronic Care Model, medical care plans, "enhanced and convenient" access to care, quantitative indicators of quality, health information technology, and feedback on performance. Payment reform was also recognized as important to the implementation of the model.

IBM and other organizations started the Patient-Centered Primary Care Collaborative in 2006 to promote the medical home model. As of 2009, its membership included "some 500 large employers, insurers, consumer groups, and doctors".

In 2007, the American Academy of Family Physicians, American Academy of Pediatrics, American College of Physicians, and American Osteopathic Association—the largest primary care physician organizations in the United States—released the *Joint Principles of the Patient-Centered Medical Home*. Defining principles included:

- Personal physician: "each patient has an ongoing relationship with a personal physician trained to provide first contact, continuous and comprehensive care."

- Physician directed medical practice: "the personal physician leads a team of individuals at the practice level who collectively take responsibility for the ongoing care of patients."

- Whole person orientation: "the personal physician is responsible for providing for all the patient's health care needs or taking responsibility for appropriately arranging care with other qualified professionals."

- Care is coordinated and/or integrated: Care is coordinated and/or integrated between complex health care systems, for example, across specialists, hospitals, home health agencies, and nursing homes, and also includes the patient's loved ones and community-based services. This goal can be attained though the utilization of registries, health information technology, and exchanges, ensuring patients receive culturally and linguistically-appropriate care.

- Quality and safety:

    o Partnerships between the patient, physicians, and their family are an integral part of the medical home. Practices are encouraged to advocate for their patients and provide compassionate quality, patient-centered care.

- o Guide decision-making rooted in evidence-based medicine and with the use of decision-support tools.

- o Physicians' voluntary engagement in performance measurements to continuously gauge quality improvement.

- o Patients are involved in decision-making and provide feedback to determine if their expectations are met.

- o Utilization of informational technology to ensure optimal patient care, performance measurement, patient education, and enhanced communication

- o At the practice level, patients and their families participate in quality improvement activities.

- Enhanced access to care is available through open scheduling, extended hours and new options for patient communication.

- Payment must "appropriately recognize the added value provided to patients who have a patient-centered medical home."

  - o Payment should reflect the time physician and non-physician staff spend doing patient-centered care management work outside the face-to-face visit.

  - o Services involved with coordination of care should be paid for.

  - o It should support measurement of quality and efficiency with the use and adoption of health information technology.

  - o Enhanced communication should be supported.

  - o It should value the time physicians spend using technology for the monitoring of clinical data.

  - o Payments for care management services should not result in deduction in payments for face-to-face service.

  - o Payment "should recognize case mix differences in the patient population being treated within the practice."

  - o It should allow physicians to share in the savings from reduced hospitalizations.

  - o It should allow for additional compensation for achieving measurable and continuous quality improvements.

A survey of 3,535 U.S. adults released in 2007 found that 27 percent of the respondents reported having "four indicators of a medical home." Furthermore, having a medical home was associated with better access to care, more preventive screenings, higher quality of care, and fewer racial and ethnic disparities.

Important developments concerning medical homes between 2008 and 2010 included:

- The Accreditation Association for Ambulatory Health Care (AAAHC) began accrediting medical homes in 2009, and is the only accrediting body to conduct on-site survey for organizations seeking Medical Home accreditation.

- The National Committee for Quality Assurance released *Physician Practice Connections– Patient-Centered Medical Home* (PPC-PCMH), a set of voluntary standards for the recognition of physician practices as medical homes.

- In answering a 2008 survey from the American Academy of Family Physicians, then-presidential candidate Barack Obama wrote "I support the concept of a patient-centered medical home" and that, as president, he would "encourage and provide appropriate payment for providers who implement the medical home model."

- The *New England Journal of Medicine* published recommendations for the success of medical homes that included increased sharing of information across health care providers, the broadening of performance measures, and the establishment of payment systems that share savings with the physicians involved.

- Guidance for patients and providers on operationalizing the "Joint Principles" was made available.

- The American Medical Association expressed support for the "Joint Principles."

- A coalition of "consumer, labor, and health care advocacy groups" released nine principles that "allow for evaluation of the medical home concept from a patient perspective."

- Initial findings of a medical home national demonstration project of the American Academy of Family Physicians were made available in 2009. A final report on the project, which began in 2006 at 36 sites, was also published in 2010.

- By 2009, 20 bills in 10 states were introduced to promote medical homes.

- In 2010, seven key health information technology domains were identified as necessary for the success of the PCMH model: telehealth, measurement of quality and efficiency, care transitions, personal health records, and, most important, registries, team care, and clinical decision support for chronic diseases.

Accreditation

The Accreditation Association for Ambulatory Health Care (AAAHC) in 2009 introduced the first accreditation program for medical homes to include an onsite survey. Unlike other quality assessment programs for medical homes, AAAHC Accreditation also mandates that PCMHs meet the Core Standards required of all ambulatory organizations seeking AAAHC Accreditation.

AAAHC standards assess PCMH providers from the perspective of the patient. The onsite survey is conducted by surveyors who are qualified professionals – physicians, registered nurses, administrators and others – who have first-hand experience with ambulatory health care organizations. The onsite survey process gives them an opportunity to directly observe the quality of patient care and the facilities in which it is delivered, review medical records and assess patient perceptions and satisfaction.

The AAAHC Accreditation Handbook for Ambulatory Health Care includes a chapter specifically devoted to medical home standards, including assessment of the following characteristics:

- Relationship, including communication, understanding and collaboration between the patient and the provider and physician-directed health care team. Where appropriate the relationship between the medical home and the patient's family or other caretakers also is assessed.

- Continuity of care, including the requirement that a significant number (more than 50 percent) of a patient's medical home visits are with the same provider/physician team. The standards also require documentation of all consultations, referrals and appointments in the clinical record; and proactively planned transitions of care (e.g. from pediatric to adult or adult to geriatric or from inpatient to outpatient to nursing home to hospice).

- Comprehensiveness of care, including preventive and wellness care, acute injury and illness care, chronic illness management and end-of-life care. Standards for the provision of appropriate patient education, self-management and community resources also are addressed.

- Accessibility, including written policies that support patient access and routine assessment of patients' perceptions and satisfaction regarding access to the medical home. Medical care must be available 24/7, 365 days a year.

- Quality, including patient care that is physician directed, the use and periodic assessment of evidence based guidelines and performance measures in delivering clinical services, and ongoing quality improvement activities.

In addition, electronic data management must be continually assessed as a tool for facilitating the Accreditation Association medical home.

AAAHC Medical Home Accreditation also requires that core standards required of all ambulatory organizations seeking AAAHC Accreditation be met, including: Standards for rights of patients; governance; administration; quality of care; quality management and improvement; clinical records and health information; infection prevention and control, and safety; and facilities and environment. Depending on the services provided, AAAHC-Accredited medical homes may also have to meet adjunct standards such as for anesthesia, surgical, pharmaceutical, pathology and medical laboratory, diagnostic and other imaging, and dental services, among others.

Certification Program

In addition to its accreditation program for medical homes, the AAAHC is conducting a pilot "Medical Home Certification" program, which includes an onsite survey to evaluate an organization against their standards for medical homes. Full accreditation requires that organizations also be evaluated against all AAAHC core standards.

Recognition Program

The National Committee for Quality Assurance's (NCQA) "Physician Practice Connections and Patient Centered Medical Home" (PPC-PCMH) Recognition Program emphasizes the systematic use of patient-centered, coordinated care management processes. It is an extension of the Physician Practice Connections Recognition Program, which was initiated in 2003 with support from organizations such as The Robert Wood Johnson Foundation, The Commonwealth Fund and Bridges to Excellence. The PPC-PCMH enhances the quality of patient care through the well known and empirically validated Wagner Chronic Care Model, which encourages the health care system to use community resources to effectively care for patients with chronic illnesses through productive interactions between activated patients and a prepared practice team. Furthermore, it recognizes practices that successfully use systematic processes and technology leading to improved quality of patient care.

With the guidance from the ACP, the AAFP, the AAP and the AOA the NCQA launched PPC-PCMH and based the program on the medical home joint principles developed by these organizations.

If practices achieve NCQA's PCMH Recognition they can take advantage of financial incentives that health plans, employers, federal and state-sponsored pilot programs offer and they may qualify for additional bonuses or payments.

In order to attain PPC-PCMH Recognition, specific elements must be met. Included in the standards are ten "must-pass" elements:

ELEMENT 1A—Access and communication processes

> The practice has written processes for scheduling appointments and communicating with patients.

ELEMENT 1B—Access and communication results

> The practice has data showing that it meets the standards in element 1A for scheduling and communicating with patients.

ELEMENT 2D—Organizing clinical data

> The practice uses electronic or paper-based charting tools to organize and document clinical information.

ELEMENT 2E—Identifying important conditions

> The practice uses an electronic or paper-based system to identify the following in the practice's patient population:

> - Most frequently seen diagnoses

> - Most important risk factors

> - Three clinically important conditions

ELEMENT 3A—Guidelines for important conditions

> The practice must implement evidence-based guidelines for the three identified clinically important conditions.

ELEMENT 4B—Self management support

> The practice works to facilitate self-management of care for patients with one of the three clinically important conditions.

ELEMENT 6A—Test tracking and follow-up

> The practice works to improve effectiveness of care by managing the timely receipt of information on all tests and results.

ELEMENT 7A—Referral tracking

> The practice seeks to improve effectiveness, timeliness and coordination of care by following through on critical consultations with other practitioners.

ELEMENT 8A—Measures of performance

> The practice measures or receives performance data by physician or across the practice regarding:

- Clinical process

- Clinical outcomes

- Service data

- Patient safety

ELEMENT 8C—Reporting to physicians

> The practice reports on its performance on the factors in Elements 8A.

Scientific Evidence

Recent peer-reviewed literature that examines the prevalence and effectiveness of medical homes includes:

- In 2007, researchers from the Centers for Disease Control and Prevention published a study involving interviews with 5400 parents; the authors concluded that continuous primary care in a medical home was associated with higher rates of vaccinations for the respondents' children.

- Schoen and colleagues (2007) surveyed adults in seven countries, using the answers to four questions to categorize the respondents as having a medical home or not. Having a medical home was associated with less difficulty accessing care after hours, improved flow of information across providers, a positive opinion about health care, fewer duplicate tests, and lower rates of medical errors.

- A review of 33 articles by Homer et al. on medical homes for children with special health care needs published in 2008 "provide moderate support for the hypothesis that medical homes provide improved health-related outcomes."

- A 2008 review by Rosenthal determined that peer-reviewed studies show "improved quality, reduced errors, and increased satisfaction when patients identify with a primary care medical home."

- In a survey of parents or legal guardians of children with special health care needs published in 2009, 47.1% of the children had a medical home, and the children with a medical home had "less delayed or forgone care and significantly fewer unmet needs for health care and family support services" than the children without a medical home.

- Reid *et al.* (2010) showed within the Group Health system in Seattle that a medical home demonstration was associated with 29% fewer emergency visits, 6% fewer hospitalizations, and total savings of $10.30 per patient per month over a twenty-one-month period (p=0.08, a result that approaches statistical significance, meaning that the difference could still be due to chance).

International Comparisons

In a study of 10 countries, the authors wrote that in most of the countries "health promotion is usually separate from acute care, so the notion of a... medical home as conceptualized in the United States... does not exist." Nevertheless, the seven-country study of Schoen et al. found that the prevalence of medical homes was highest in New Zealand (61%) and lowest in Germany (45%).

Controversy

Comparison with "Gatekeeper" Models

Some suggest that the medical home mimics the managed care "gatekeeper" models historically employed by HMOs; however, there are important distinctions between care coordination in the medical home and the "gatekeeper" model. In the medical home, the patient has open access to see whatever physician they choose. No referral or permission is required. The personal physician of choice, who has comprehensive knowledge of the patient's medical conditions, facilitates and provides information to subspecialists involved in the care of the patient. The gatekeeper model placed more financial risk on the physicians resulting in rewards for less care. The medical home puts emphasis on medical management rewarding quality patient-centered care.

Organizations Criticizing the Model

The medical home model has its critics, including the following major organizations:

- The American College of Emergency Physicians expresses cautions such as "a shifting of financial and other resources to support the PCMH model could have adverse effects on sectors of the health care system" and "there should be proven value in health care outcomes for patients and reduced costs to the health care system before there is widespread implementation of this model."

- The American Optometric Association is concerned that medical homes "may restrict access to eye and vision care" and requests "that optometry be recognized as a principal provider of eye and vision care services within the PCMH"

- The American Psychological Association states that Congress should ensure that "careful consideration is paid to the role of psychologists and non-physician providers in the medical home model, which should be more appropriately named the 'health home model'."

Costs

Clinics compliant with principles of the patient-centered medical home may be associated with increase operating costs.

Ongoing Medical Home Projects

One notable implementation of medical homes has been Community Care of North Carolina (CCNC), which was started under the name "Carolina Access" in the early 1990s. CCNC consists of 14 community health networks that link approximately 750,000 Medicaid patients to medical homes. It is funded by North Carolina's Medicaid office, which pays $3 per member per month to networks and $2.50 per member per month to physicians. CCNC is reported to have improved healthcare for patients with asthma and diabetes. Non-peer-reviewed analyses cited in a peer-reviewed article suggested that CCNC saved North Carolina $60 million in fiscal year 2003 and $161 million in fiscal year 2006. However, an independent analysis asserted that CCNC cost the state over $400 million in 2006 instead of producing savings. More recent analyses show that the program improved the quality of care for asthma and diabetes patients significantly, reducing emergency department and hospital use that produced savings of $150 million in 2007 alone.

The Rhode Island Chronic Care Sustainability Initiative (CSI-RI) is a community-wide collaborative effort convened in 2006 by the Office of the Health Insurance Commissioner to develop a sustainable model of primary care that will improve the care of chronic disease and lead to better overall health outcomes for Rhode Islanders. CSI-RI is focused on improving the delivery of chronic illness care and supporting and sustaining primary care in the state of Rhode Island through the development and implementation of the patient-centered medical home. The CSI-RI Medical Home demonstration officially launched in October 2008 with 5 primary care practices and was expanded in April 2010 to include an additional 8 sites. Thirteen primary care sites, 66 providers, 39 Family Medicine residents, 68,000 patients (46,000 covered lives), and all Rhode Island payers are participating in the demonstration. Further, its selection to participate in the Centers for Medicare and Medicaid Services' Multi-Payer Advanced Primary Care Practice demonstration, CSI-RI is one few medical home demonstrations in the nation with virtually 100% payer participation. Since the start of the demonstration, CSI-RI sites have implemented a series of delivery system reforms in their practices, aimed at becoming patient-centered medical homes, and in turn receive a supplemental per-member-per-month payment from all of Rhode Island's insurers. Each participating practice site also receives funding from participating payers for an on-site nurse care manager, who can work with all patients in the practice, regardless of insurance type or status. All 5 original pilot sites achieved NCQA level 1 PPC-PCMH recognition in 2009, and all 8 expansion sites achieved at least level 1 PPC-PCMH recognition in 2010. As of December 2010, all of the pilot sites and two of the expansion sites have been recognized by NCQA as level 3 patient-centered medical homes.

Projects Evaluating Medical Home Concepts

The Agency for Healthcare Research and Quality offers grants to primary care practices in order for them to become patient-centered medical homes. The grants are designed to increase the evidence base for these types of transformations.

As of December 31, 2009, there were at least 26 pilot projects involving medical homes with external payment reform being conducted in 18 states. These pilots included over 14,000 physicians caring for nearly 5 million patients. The projects are evaluating factors such as clinical quality, cost, patient experience/satisfaction, and provider experience/satisfaction. Some of the projects underway are:

- Division B, Section 204 of the *Tax Relief and Health Care Act of 2006* outlined a Medicare medical home demonstration project. This three-year project will involve care management reimbursement and incentive payments to physicians in 400 practices in 8 sites. It will evaluate the health and economic benefits of providing "targeted, accessible, continuous and coordinated, family-centered care to high-need populations." As of July 2009, however, the project had not yet started recruiting practices.

- In 2008, CIGNA and Dartmouth-Hitchcock announced they had launched a pilot program in New Hampshire with 391 primary care providers.

- A UnitedHealth Group medical home pilot in Arizona involving 7,000 patients and 7 medical groups began in 2009 and is scheduled to end in 2011.

- The state of Maine provided $500,000 in 2009 for a pilot project in 26 practices.

- The New Jersey Academy of Family Physicians and Horizon Blue Cross and Blue Shield of New Jersey implemented a pilot project in March 2009. This project is ongoing and involves more than 60 primary care practice sites and 165 primary care physicians. Specialties include family medicine/practice, internal medicine and multi-specialties in which 50% or more of the care provided is primary care.

- The Texas Medical Home Initiative, a multi-stakeholder primary-care driven organization, has launched a two-year pilot involving 7 primary care practices in North and East Texas. This project involves 45 physicians and 75,000 patients. Services to the practices include practice coaching, a patient registry system, assistance with developing practice agreements with specialty practices to build the "medical neighborhood".

In 2006, TransforMED announced the launch of the National Demonstration Project aimed at transforming the way primary care is delivered in our country. The practice redesign initiative, funded by the AAFP, ran from June 2006 to May 2008. It was the first and largest "proof-of-concept" project to determine empirically whether the TransforMED Patient-Centered Medical Home model of care could be implemented successfully and sustained in today's health care environment. More specifically, the project served as a learning lab to gain better insight into the kinds of hands-on technical support family physicians want and need to implement the PCMH model of care. Learn more about National Demonstration Project

Between 2002 and 2006, Group Health Cooperative made reforms to increase efficiency and access at 20 primary care clinics in western Washington. These reforms had an adverse impact, increasing physician workload, fatigue, and turnover. Negative trends in quality of care and utilization also appeared. As a result, the Group Health Research Institute developed a patient-centered medical home model in one of the clinics. By increasing staff, patient outreach and care management, the clinic reduced emergency department visits and improved patient perceptions of care quality.

The Role of PCMH and Accountable Care Organizations (ACO) in the Coordination of Patient Care

There are four core functions of primary care as conceptualized by Barbara Starfield and the Institute of Medicine. These four core functions consist of providing "accessible, comprehensive, longitudinal, and coordinated care in the context of families and community".

In the PCMH model, the integration of diverse services that a patient may need is encouraged. This integration which also involves the patient in interpreting the streams of information and working together to find a plan that fits with the patient's values and preferences is under-recognized and under-appreciated.

Appropriate coordinated care depends on the patient or the population of patients and to a large extent, the complexity of their needs. The challenges involved with facilitating the delivery of care increases as the complexity of their needs increase. These complexities include chronic or acute health conditions, the social vulnerability of the patient, and the environment of the patient including the number of providers involved in their care. Other factors that may play a role in the patient's coordination of care include their preferences and their ability to organize their own care. The increases in complexity may overwhelm informal coordinating functions requiring a care team that can explicitly provide coordinated care and assume responsibility for the coordination of a particular patient's care.

According to the ACO, care coordination achieves two critical objectives—high-quality and high-value care. ACOs can build on the coordinated care provided by the PCMHs and ensure and incentivize communications between teams of providers that operate in various settings. ACOs can facilitate transitions and align the resources needed to meet the clinical and coordinated care needs of the population. They can develop and support systems for the coordination of care of patients in non-ambulatory care settings. Furthermore, they can monitor health information systems and the timeliness and completeness of information transactions between primary care physicians and specialists. The tracking of this information can be used to incentivize higher levels of responsiveness and collaborations.

Ambulatory Care

Ambulatory care or outpatient care is medical care provided on an outpatient basis, including diagnosis, observation, consultation, treatment, intervention, and rehabilitation services. This care can include advanced medical technology and procedures even when provided outside of hospitals.

Ambulatory care sensitive conditions (ACSC) are health conditions where appropriate ambulatory care prevents or reduces the need for hospital admission (or *inpatient* care), such as diabetes or chronic obstructive pulmonary disease.

Many Medical Investigations and treatments for acute and chronic illnesses and preventive health care can be performed on an ambulatory basis, including minor surgical and medical procedures, most types of dental services, dermatology services, and many types of diagnostic procedures (e.g. blood tests, X-rays, endoscopy and biopsy procedures of superficial organs). Other types of ambulatory care services include emergency visits, rehabilitation visits, and in some cases telephone consultations.

Ambulatory care services represent the most significant contributor to increasing hospital expenditures and to the performance of the health care system in most countries, including most developing countries.

Settings

Health care organizations use different ways to define the nature of care provided as "ambulatory" versus inpatient or other types of care.

Sites where ambulatory care can be delivered include:

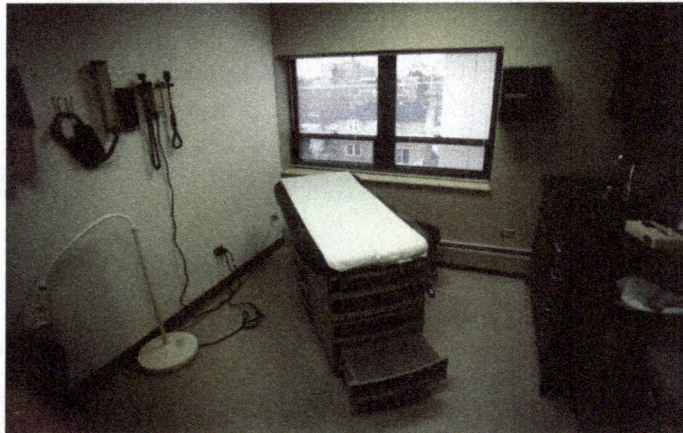

An examination room in a doctor's office.

- Doctor's surgeries (known as doctor's offices in American English): This is the most common site for the delivery of ambulatory care in many countries, and usually consists of a physician's visit. Physicians of many specialties deliver ambulatory care. These physicians include specialists in family medicine, internal medicine, obstetrics, gynaecology, cardiology, gastroenterology, endocrinology, ophthalmology, and dermatology.

- Clinics: Including ambulatory care clinics, polyclinics, ambulatory surgery centers, and urgent care centers.

    o   In the United States, the Urgent Care Association of America (UCAOA) estimates that over 15,000 urgent care centers deliver urgent care services. These centers are designed to evaluate and treat conditions that are not severe enough to require treatment in a hospital emergency department but still require treatment beyond normal physician office hours or before a physician appointment is available.

  o   In Russia and other countries of the former Soviet Union, Feldsher health stations are the main site for ambulatory care in rural areas.

- Hospitals: Including emergency departments and other hospital-based services such as same day surgery services and mental health services.

  o   Hospital emergency departments: Some visits to emergency departments result in hospital admission, so these would be considered emergency medicine visits rather than ambulatory care. Most visits to hospital emergency departments, however, do not require hospital admission.

- Non-medical institution-based settings: Including school and prison health; vision, dental and pharmaceutical care.

- Non-institution settings: For example, mass childhood immunization campaigns using community health workers.

Conditions

Ambulatory care sensitive conditions (ACSC) are illnesses or health conditions where appropriate ambulatory care prevents or reduces the need for hospital admission. Appropriate care for an ACSC can include one or more planned revisits to settings of ambulatory care for follow-up, such as when a patient is continuously monitored or otherwise advised to return when (or if) symptoms appear or reappear.

Relatively common ACSC include:

• asthma	• congestive heart failure
• angina	• epilepsy
• diabetes (complications)	• influenza, pneumonia and other vaccine-preventable diseases
• chronic obstructive pulmonary disease	• tuberculosis
• pelvic inflammatory disease	• iron deficiency anemia
• hypertension	• urinary tract infections
• chronic pain, pain management	• cellulitis
• gastroenteritis	• dental conditions.
• gangrene	
• ear-nose-throat (ENT) infections	

Hospitalization for an ACSC is considered to be a measure of access to appropriate primary health care, including preventive and disease management services. While not all admissions for these conditions are avoidable, appropriate ambulatory care could help prevent their onset, control an acute episode, or manage a chronic disease or condition.: For Medicaid-covered and uninsured U.S. hospital stays in 2012, six of the top ten diagnoses were ambulatory care sensitive conditions.

Community Health Center

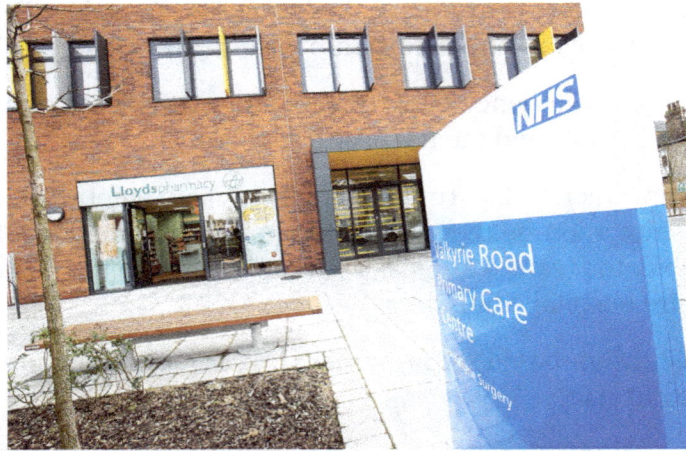

An NHS health centre in the United Kingdom (Murphy Philipps Architects)

A healthcare center, health center, or community health center is one of a network of clinics staffed by a group of general practitioners and nurses providing healthcare services to people in a certain area. Typical services covered are family practice and dental care, but some clinics have expanded greatly and can include internal medicine, pediatric, women's care, family planning, pharmacy, optometry, lab, and more. In countries with universal healthcare, most people use the healthcare centers. In countries without universal healthcare, the clients include the uninsured, underinsured, low-income or those living in areas where little access to primary health care is available.

Community Health Centres by Country

Canada

Community Health Centers (CHCs) have existed in Ontario for more than 40 years. Most CHC's consist of an interdisciplinary team of health care providers using electronic health records.

In Quebec, local community services centres known by their French acronym, CLSC, offer routine health and social services, including consultations with general practitioners with and without an appointment.

China

In China there are, as of 2011, 32,812 community health centers and 37,374 township health centers.

Portugal

The health center (Portuguese: *centro de saúde*) was the basic community primary healthcare unit of the National Health Service of Portugal, as well as acting as the local public health authority. Usually, each health center covered the area of one of the Portuguese municipalities, but municipalities with over than 15 000 habitants could be covered by more than one of these centers.

Health centers were staffed with general practitioners, public health physicians, nurses, social workers and administrative personnel.

In 2008, the more than 300 health centers were aggregated into around 70 health center groups (*agrupamentos de centros de saúde*) or ACES. Each ACES includes several family and personalized healthcare units, these being now the basic primary health care providers of the Portuguese National Health Service. Besides family health care services, the ACES also include public health, community health and other specialized units, as well as basic medical emergency services.

Some of the ACES were grouped with hospital units into experimental local health units (*unidades locais de saúde*) or ULS. The ULS are intended to increase the coordination between the primary and the secondary healthcare, through both of these services being provided by the same health unit.

United Kingdom

Lord Dawson of Penn was commissioned by Lord Addison to produce a report on "schemes requisite for the systematised provision of such forms of medical and allied services as should... be available for the inhabitants of a given area". The Interim Report on the Future Provision of Medical and Allied Services was produced in 1920, though no further report ever appeared. The report laid down detailed plans for a network of Primary and Secondary Health Centres, together with detailed architectural drawings of different sorts of centres. By 1939 the term health centre was widely used to refer to new buildings housing local health authority services. The Dawson report was very influential in debates about the National Health Service when it was set up in 1948, but few centres were built because "it was not practicable for local authorities to establish health centres without the full compliance of general practitioners" - which was not forthcoming. Far more attention and resources were devoted to hospital services than to primary care. From 1948 to 1974 local authorities were responsible for the building of health centres.

A well known centre was opened at Woodberry Down in October 1952. It had provision for 6 GPs, 2 dentists, a pharmacist and two nurses. It cost about £163,000, which included the cost of a day nursery and child guidance clinic. This was regarded as extravagant and used as an excuse by critics for not building more. Harlow, where 4 centres were built by the new town corporation, was the only community in Britain served exclusively by doctors working from health centres.

The few centres that were built "functioned as isolated islands in a sea of General Practitioners generally indifferent to their success". There were later calls to establish a network of centres to include not only GPs but also dentists and diagnostic facilities. In 1965 there were only 30 health centres in England and Wales, and 3 in Scotland. By 1974 there were 566 in England, 29 in Wales and 59 in Scotland. After the National Health Service Reorganisation Act 1973, responsibility for promoting health centres was transferred to Area Health Authorities and there were renewed calls to establish more Health Centres. It was suggested that these centres could arrange alternative medical care for patients "when their doctor is off duty, or for emergency calls when he is engaged elsewhere".

Lord Darzi set up a network of Polyclinics in England when he was a minister in 2008. These clinics had some features in common with earlier proposals for health centres, but shared with them considerable resistance from GPs.

United States

In the U.S., Community Health Centers (CHCs) are neighborhood health centers generally serving Medically Underserved Areas (MUAs) which includes persons who are uninsured, underinsured, low-income or those living in areas where little access to primary health care is available. Largely federally and locally funded, some health clinics are modernized with new equipment and electronic medical records. In 2006, the National Association of Community Health Centers implemented a model for offering free, rapid HIV testing to all patients between the ages of 13 and 64 during routine primary medical and dental care visits.

Medically Underserved Areas/Populations are areas or populations designated by the Health Resources and Services Administration (HRSA) as having: too few primary care providers, high infant mortality, high poverty and/or high elderly population. Health Professional Shortage Areas (HPSAs) are designated by HRSA as having shortages of primary medical care, dental or mental health providers and may be geographic (a county or service area), demographic (low income population) or institutional (comprehensive health center, federally qualified health center or other public facility).

Community Therapeutic Care

Community Therapeutic Care is a new approach to dealing with acute malnutrition.

Community-based Therapeutic Care (CTC) was developed to improve the coverage and impact of selective feeding programs for the treatment of acute malnutrition. Its central innovation is to provide therapeutic feeding in the home.

Before the development of CTC, the traditional way of treating malnutrition was through therapeutic feeding centers: large centers where patients are admitted for an average of 30 days. Carers of malnourished children often have to travel long distances to access these centers, many having to leave the rest of their children at home for three weeks or longer.

Until recently, therapeutic feeding centers, that require long inpatient stays, have been the only accepted mode of treatment for severe acute malnutrition. CTC programmes treat the majority of these cases at home and aim to restrict inpatient care to only those suffering from acute malnutrition with medical complications. They use decentralised networks of outpatient treatment sites to provide a take-home food ration known as Ready-to-Use Therapeutic Food (RUTF) along with routine medicines.

By providing easy access and reducing the opportunity costs associated with enrollment in a therapeutic feeding programme, the CTC model increases the coverage and impact of humanitarian feeding interventions.

During the early years, the focus of CTC was on developing and demonstrating a model that can achieve rapid and widespread impact on the mortality and morbidity of children under five in emergency situations. Data from CTC programmes demonstrate that CTC can achieve very high coverage and excellent recovery rates. CTC has gained widespread acceptance in the humanitarian sector and is now the preferred model for selective feeding in emergency contexts.

Nurse-managed Health Center

A nurse-managed health center provides health care services in medically underserved rural and urban areas in the United States where there is limited access to health care. Nurse-managed health centers provide health care to thousands of uninsured and underinsured people every year. Nurse-managed health centers are usually affiliated with nursing schools, universities, and/or independent non-profit organizations. Managed by advanced practice nurses, nurse-managed health centers provide health care to vulnerable communities using a nursing model.

Overview

The first nurse-managed health center was created at Arizona State University over 25 years ago, and it is still in existence today. Now, there are approximately 250 Nurse-Managed Health Centers in the United States, located in 39 states and the District of Columbia. Currently, Philadelphia has more Nurse-Managed Health Centers than any other city in the United States.

Nurse-managed health centers serve populations that are demographically similar to those served by Federally Qualified Health Centers (FQHCs). In some cases, Nurse-Managed Health Centers are FQHCs. Nurse-Managed Health Centers tend to be located in or near low-income communities. Over half of the patients seen at Nurse-Managed Health Centers are females who come from racial/ethnic minority populations and are likely to have experienced health disparities.

Nurse-Managed Health Centers are managed and staffed by advanced practice nurses, including nurse practitioners. In some Nurse-Managed Health Centers, nurses collaborate with physicians to provide care. In other Nurse-Managed Health Centers, nurses work independently.

The National Nursing Centers Consortium is the national nonprofit organization that works to advance nurse-led health care through policy, consultation, programs and applied research to reduce health disparities and meet people's primary care and wellness needs. The nation's 250 nurse-managed health clinics reduce health disparities by providing high quality comprehensive primary health care, health promotion and disease prevention services to uninsured, under-insured and vulnerable patients in rural, urban and suburban communities.

Services Provided

Many Nurse-Managed Health Centers provide a full range of primary care services including preventive care, similar to services provided by primary care physicians. Research has shown, however, that nurses in Nurse Managed Health Centers spend more time with patients and include more preventive care than physicians. Some Nurse-Managed Health Centers also provide behavioral health services, including family and couples therapy. In addition, all Nurse-Managed Health Centers provide health promotion, wellness, and disease management services.

Nurse-Managed Health Centers also focus on preventive health care, especially regarding certain chronic conditions like asthma, hypertension, diabetes, and obesity. This focus on preventative, holistic health care has been shown to reduce emergency room usage and decrease the length of hospital stays among Nurse-Managed Health Center patients.

Representation

The National Nursing Centers Consortium (NNCC) is a 501(c)3 and is the national organization supporting and advocating on behalf of NMHCs and nurse-led care. NNCC currently represents more than 250 NMHCs throughout the nation. They advocate for policy initiatives at the state and federal level on behalf of nurse practitioners scope of practice and also increased funding for NMHCs. NNCC is headquartered in Philadelphia, PA

Telehealth

Telehealth involves the distribution of health-related services and information. Distribution is via electronic information and telecommunication technologies. It allows long distance patient/clinician contact and care, advice, reminders, education, intervention, monitoring and remote admissions. As well as provider distance-learning; meetings, supervision, and presentations between practitioners; online information and health data management and healthcare system integration. Telehealth could include two clinicians discussing a case over video conference; a robotic surgery occurring through remote access; physical therapy done via digital monitoring instruments, live feed and application combinations; tests being forwarded between facilities for interpretation by a higher specialist; home monitoring through continuous sending of patient health data; client to practitioner online conference; or even videophone interpretation during a consult.

As the population grows and ages, and medical advances are made which prolong life, demands increase on the healthcare system. Healthcare providers are also being asked to do more, with no increase in funding, or are encouraged to move to new models of funding and care such as patient-centred or outcomes based, rather than fee-for-service. Some specific health professions already have a shortage (i.e. Speech-language pathologists). When rural settings, lack of transport, lack of mobility (i.e. In the elderly or disabled), decreased funding or lack of staffing restrict access to care, telehealth can bridge the gap.

Telehealth Versus Telemedicine

Telehealth is sometimes discussed interchangeably with telemedicine. The Health Resources and Services Administration (HRSA) distinguishes telehealth from telemedicine in its scope. According to HRSA, telemedicine only describes remote clinical services; such as diagnosis and monitoring, while telehealth includes preventative, promotive and curative care delivery. This includes the above-mentioned non-clinical applications like administration and provider education which make telehealth the preferred modern terminology.

History

The development and history of telehealth or telemedicine (terms used interchangeably in literature) is deeply rooted in the history and development in not only technology but also society itself. Humans have long sought to relay important messages through torches, optical telegraphy, electroscopes, and wireless transmission. In the 21st century, with the advent of the internet, portable devices and other such digital devices are taking a transformative role in healthcare and its delivery.

Earliest Instances

Although, traditional medicine relies on in-person care, the need and want for remote care has existed from the Roman and pre-Hippocratic periods in antiquity. The elderly and infirm who could not visit temples for medical care sent representatives to convey information on symptoms and bring home a diagnosis as well as treatment. In Africa, villagers would use smoke signals to warn neighbouring villages of disease outbreak. The beginnings of telehealth have existed through primitive forms of communication and technology.

1800s to Early 1900s

As technology developed and wired communication became increasingly commonplace, the ideas surround telehealth began emerging. The earliest telehealth encounter can be traced to Alexander Graham Bell in 1876, when he used his early telephone as a means of getting help from his assistant Mr Watson after he spilt acid on his trousers. Another instance of early telehealth, specifically telemedicine was reported in *The Lancet* in 1879. An anonymous writer described a case where a doctor successfully diagnosed a child over the telephone in the middle of the night. This Lancet issue, also further discussed the potential of Remote Patient Care in order to avoid unnecessary house visits, which were part of routine health care during the 1800s. Other instances of telehealth during this period came from the American Civil War, during which telegraphs were used to deliver mortality lists and medical care to soldiers.

From the late 1800s to the early 1900s the early foundations of wireless communication were laid down. Radios provided an easier and near instantaneous form of communication. The use of radio to deliver healthcare became accepted for remote areas. The Royal Flying Doctor Service of Australia is an example of the early adoption of radios in telehealth.

Mid-1900s to 1980s

It was during the mid-1900s well into the 1980s that a lot of the momentum and foundations of telehealth were founded. When the American National Aeronautics and Space Administration (NASA), began plans to send astronauts into space, the need for Telemedicine became all too clear. In order to monitor their astronauts in space, telemedicine capabilities were built into the spacecraft as well as the first spacesuits. Additionally, during this period, telehealth and Telemedicine were promoted in different countries especially the United States. Different projects were funded across North America and Canada in order to realise the exciting potential of this new innovation.

In 1964, the Nebraska Psychiatric Institute began using television links to form two-way communication with the Norfolk State Hospital which was 112 miles away for the education and consultation purposes between clinicians in the two locations. The Logan International Airport in Boston established in-house medical stations in 1967. These stations were linked to Massachusetts General Hospital. Clinicians at the hospital would provide consultation services to patients who were at the airport. Consultations were achieved through microwave audio as well as video links.

In 1972, there was a key emphasis on telemedicine so much so that the Department of Health, Education and Welfare in the United States approved funding for seven telemedicine projects across different states. This funding was renewed and two further projects were funded the following year.

1980s to 1990s – maturation and Renaissance

Although the excitement of telehealth and telemedicine remained, enthusiasm waned in the 1980s. Telehealth projects underway before and during the 1980s would take off but fail to proliferate mainstream healthcare. This put a halt on various projects and reduced opportunities for funding. As a result, this period of telehealth history is called the "maturation" stage and made way for sustainable growth.

Sustained growth happened most notably in North America. Although State funding was beginning to run low, different hospitals in various states began to launch their own telehealth initiatives. Additionally, NASA started experimenting with their ATS-3 satellite. Eventually, NASA started their SateLife/HealthNet programme which tried to increase the health services connectivity in developing countries.

The combination of sustained growth, the advent of the internet and the increasing adoption of ICT in traditional methods of care spurred the revival or "renaissance" of telehealth into the early 2000s and onwards.

2000s and Onward

The early 2000s were characterised by accelerated development in both science and technology. The early adoption of technology in society made way for widespread adoption in society. The diffusion of portable devices like laptops and mobile devices in everyday life made ideas surrounding telehealth more plausible. This continuing trend of better and innovative technology in homes, schools and organisations is contributing to the growing research in telehealth. Telehealth is no longer bound within the realms of telemedicine but has expanded itself to promotion, prevention and education.

Methods and Modalities

Telehealth requires a strong, reliable broadband connection. The broadband signal transmission infrastructure includes wires, cables, microwaves and optic fibre, which must be maintained for the provision of telehealth services. The better the connection (bandwidth quality), the more data can be sent and received. Historically this has priced providers or patients out of the service, but as the infrastructure improves and becomes more accessible, telehealth usage can grow.

When a healthcare service decides to provide telehealth to its patients, there are steps to consider, besides just whether the above resources are available. A needs assessment is the best way to start, which includes assessing the access the community currently has to the proposed specialists and care, whether the organisation currently has underutilized equipment which will make them useful to the area they are trying to service, and the hardships they are trying to improve by providing the access to their intended community (i.e. Travel time, costs, time off work). A service then needs to consider potential collaborators. Other services may exist in the area with similar goals who could be joined to provide a more holistic service, and/or they may already have telehealth resources available. The more services involved, the easier to spread the cost of IT, training, workflow changes and improve buy-in from clients. Services need to have the patience to wait for the accrued benefits of providing their telehealth service and cannot necessarily expect community-wide changes reflected straight away.

Once the need for a Telehealth service is established, delivery can come within four distinct domains. They are live video (synchronous), store-and-forward (asynchronous), remote patient monitoring, and mobile health. Live video involves a real-time two-way interaction, such as patient/caregiver-provider or provider-provider, over a digital (i.e. broadband) connection. This often is used to substitute a face to face meeting such as consults, and saves time and cost in travel. Store-and-forward is when data is collected, recorded, and then sent on to a provider. For example, a patient's' digital health history file including x-rays and notes, being securely transmitted electronically to evaluate the current case. Remote patient monitoring includes patients' medical and health data being collected and transferred to a provider elsewhere who can continue to monitor the data and any changes that may occur. This may best suit cases that require ongoing care such as rehabilitation, chronic care, or elderly clients trying to stay in the community in their own homes as opposed to a care facility. Mobile health includes any health information, such as education, monitoring and care, that is present on and supported by mobile communication devices such as cell phones or tablet computers. This might include an application, or text messaging services like appointment reminders or public health warning systems.

Major Developments

In Policy

Telehealth is a modern form of health care delivery. Telehealth breaks away from traditional health care delivery by using modern telecommunication systems including wireless communication methods. Traditional health is legislated through policy to ensure the safety of medical practitioners and patients. Consequently, since telehealth is a new form of health care delivery that is now gathering momentum in the health sector, many organizations have started to legislate the use of telehealth into policy. In New Zealand, the Medical Council has a statement about telehealth on their website. This illustrates that the medical council has foreseen the importance that telehealth will have on the health system and have started to introduce telehealth legislation to practitioners along with government.

Transition to Mainstream

Traditional use of telehealth services has been for specialist treatment. However, there has been a paradigm shift and telehealth is no longer considered a specialist service. This development has ensured that many access barriers are eliminated, as medical professionals are able to use wireless communication technologies to deliver health care. This is evident in rural communities. For individuals living in rural communities, specialist care can be some distance away, particularly in the next major city. Telehealth eliminates this barrier, as health professionals are able to conduct a medical consultation through the use of wireless communication technologies. However, this process is dependent on both parties having Internet access.

Telehealth allows the patient to be monitored between physician office visits which can improve patient health. Telehealth also allows patients to access expertise which is not available in their local area. This remote patient monitoring ability enables patients to stay at home longer and helps avoid unnecessary hospital time. In the long-term, this could potentially result in less burdening of the healthcare system and consumption of resources.

Technology Advancement

The technological advancement of wireless communication devices is a major development in telehealth. This allows patients to self-monitor their health conditions and to not rely as much on health care professionals. Furthermore, patients are more willing to stay on their treatment plans as they are more invested and included in the process, decision-making is shared. Technological advancement also means that health care professionals are able to use better technologies to treat patients for example in surgery. Technological developments in telehealth are essential to improve health care, especially the delivery of healthcare services, as resources are finite along with an ageing population that is living longer.

Major Implications and Impacts

Telehealth allows multiple, different disciplines to merge and deliver a much more uniform level of care using the efficiency and accessibility of everyday technology. As telehealth proliferates mainstream healthcare and challenges notions of traditional healthcare delivery, different populations are starting to experience better quality, access and personalised care in their lives.

Health Promotion

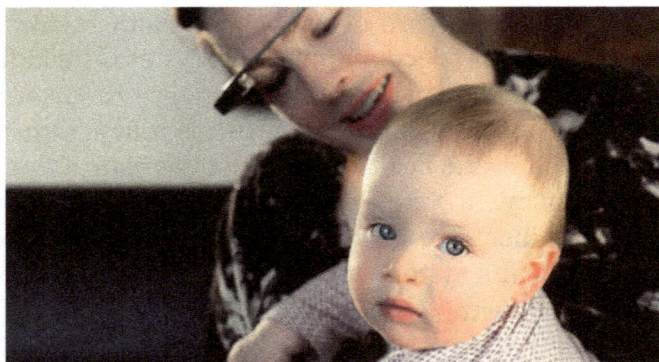

Baby Eve with Georgia for the Breastfeeding Support Project

Telehealth can also increase health promotion efforts. These efforts can now be more personalised to the target population and professionals can extend their help into homes or private and safe environments in which patients of individuals can practice, ask and gain health information. Health promotion using telehealth has become increasingly popular in underdeveloped countries where there are very poor physical resources available. There has been a particular push toward mHealth applications as many areas, even underdeveloped ones have mobile phone coverage.

In developed countries, health promotion efforts using telehealth have been met with some success. The Australian hands-free breastfeeding Google Glass application reported promising results in 2014. This application made in collaboration with the Australian Breastfeeding Association and a tech startup called Small World Social, helped new mothers learn how to breastfeed. Breastfeeding is beneficial to infant health and maternal health and is recommended by the World Health Organisation and health organisations all over the world. Widespread breastfeeding can prevent 820,000 infant deaths globally but the practice is often stopped prematurely or intents to do are disrupted due to lack of social support, know-how or other factors. This application gave mother's hands-free information on breastfeeding, instructions on how to breastfeed and also had an option to call a lactation consultant over Google Hangout. When the trial ended, all participants were reported to be confident in breastfeeding.

Health Care Quality

Theoretically, the whole health system stands to benefit from telehealth. In a UK telehealth trial done in 2011, it was reported that the cost of health could be dramatically reduced with the use of telehealth monitoring. The usual cost of in-vitro fertilization (IVF) per cycle would be around $15,000, with telehealth it was reduced to $800 per patient. In Alaska the Federal Health Care Access Network which connects 3,000 healthcare providers to communities, engaged in 160,000 telehealth consultations from 2001 and saved the state $8.5 million in travel costs for just Medicaid patients. There are indications telehealth consumes fewer resources and requires fewer people to operate it with shorter training periods to implement initiatives.

However, whether or not the standard of health care quality is increasing is quite debatable, with literature refuting such claims. Research is increasingly reporting that clinicians find the process difficult and complex to deal with. Furthermore, there are concerns around informed consent, legality issues as well as legislative issues. Although health care may become affordable with the help of technology, whether or not this care will be "good" is the issue.

Nonclinical Uses

- Distance education including continuing medical education, grand rounds, and patient education

- administrative uses including meetings among telehealth networks, supervision, and presentations

- research on telehealth

- online information and health data management

- healthcare system integration

- asset identification, listing, and patient to asset matching, and movement

- overall healthcare system management

- patient movement and remote admission

Limitations and Restrictions

While many branches of medicine have wanted to fully embrace telehealth for a long time, there are certain risks and barriers which bar the full amalgamation of telehealth into best practice. For a start, it is dubious as to whether a practitioner can fully leave the "hands-on" experience behind. Although it is predicted that telehealth will replace many consultations and other health interactions, it cannot yet fully replace a physical examination, this is particularly so in diagnostics, rehabilitation or mental health.

The benefits posed by telehealth challenge the normative means of healthcare delivery set in both legislation and practice. Therefore, the growing prominence of telehealth is starting to underscore the need for updated regulations, guidelines and legislation which reflect the current and future trends of healthcare practices. Telehealth enables timely and flexible care to patients wherever they may be; although this is a benefit, it also poses threats to privacy, safety, medical licensing and reimbursement. When a clinician and patient are in different locations, it is difficult to determine which laws apply to the context. Once healthcare crosses borders different state bodies are involved in order to regulate and maintain the level of care that is warranted to the patient or telehealth consumer. As it stands, telehealth is complex with many grey areas when put into practice especially as it crosses borders. This effectively limits the potential benefits of telehealth.

An example of these limitations include the current American reimbursement infrastructure, where Medicare will reimburse for telehealth services only when a patient is living in an area where specialists are in shortage, or in particular rural counties. The area is defined by whether it is a medical facility as opposed to a patient's' home. The site that the practitioner is in, however, is unrestricted. Medicare will only reimburse live video (synchronous) type services, not store-and-forward, mhealth or remote patient monitoring (if it does not involve live-video). Some insurers currently will reimburse telehealth, but not all yet. So providers and patients must go to the extra effort of finding the correct insurers before continuing. Again in America, states generally tend to require that clinicians are licensed to practice in the surgery' state, therefore they can only provide their service if licensed in an area that they do not live in themselves.

More specific and widely reaching laws, legislations and regulations will have to evolve with the technology. They will have to be fully agreed upon, for example, will all clinicians need full licensing in every community they provide telehealth services too, or could there be a limited use telehealth licence? Would the limited use licence cover all potential telehealth interventions, or only some? Who would be responsible if an emergency was occurring and the practitioner could not provide immediate help – would someone else have to be in the room with the patient at all consult times? Which state, city or country would the law apply in when a breach or malpractice occurred?

A major legal action prompt in telehealth thus far has been issues surrounding online prescribing and whether an appropriate clinician-patient relationship can be established online to make prescribing safe, making this an area that requires particular scrutiny. It may be required that the practitioner and patient involved must meet in person at least once before online prescribing can occur, or that at least a live-video conference must occur, not just impersonal questionnaires or surveys to determine need.

Ethical Issues

Informed consent is another issue – should the patient give informed consent to receive online care before it starts? Or will it be implied if it is care that can only practically be given over distance? When telehealth includes the possibility for technical problems such as transmission errors or security breaches or storage which impact on ability to communicate, it may be wise to obtain informed consent in person first, as well as having backup options for when technical issues occur. In person, a patient can see who is involved in their care (namely themselves and their clinician in a consult), but online there will be other involved such as the technology providers, therefore consent may need to involve disclosure of anyone involved in the transmission of the information and the security that will keep their information private, and any legal malpractice cases may need to involve all of those involved as opposed to what would usually just be the practitioner.

The State of the Market

The rate of adoption of telehealth services in any jurisdiction is frequently influenced by factors such as the adequacy and cost of existing conventional health services in meeting patient needs; the policies of governments and/or insurers with respect to coverage and payment for telehealth services; and medical licensing requirements that may inhibit or deter the provision of telehealth second opinions or primary consultations by physicians.

Projections for the growth of the telehealth market are optimistic, and much of this optimism is predicated upon the increasing demand for remote medical care. According to a recent survey, nearly three-quarters of U.S. consumers say they would use telehealth. At present, several major companies along with a bevvy of startups are working to develop a leading presence in the field.

In the UK, the Government's Care Services minister, Paul Burstow, has stated that telehealth and telecare would be extended over the next five years (2012–2017) to reach three million people.

Telehomecare

Telehomecare (THC) is a subfield within telehealth. It involves the delivery of healthcare services to patients at home through the use of telecommunications technologies, which enable the interaction of voice, video, and health-related data. The management of care is done from an external site by a healthcare professional.

It is often interchanged with remote patient monitoring; however, telehomecare is not strictly patient monitoring because it incorporates a range of health care delivery through education, emotional and social support, information dissemination, and self-care help and suggestions. The implementation of THC helps to better manage patients with chronic health conditions such as heart disease, COPD, diabetes, etc., and less visits to primary health care services can result. THC increases the accessibility to health care services especially as the need for homecare rises with the aging population. Additionally, THC can help create networks of services between hospitals and primary care providers, thereby allowing patients better access to services. In addition to improving management of chronic conditions and increasing access to healthcare, THC is believed to reduce costs of healthcare.

THC technology is designed to meet the needs of a range of patients. There can be patients requiring minimal monitoring or very sophisticated monitoring. A system can consist of a small unit to which one or more peripheral devices are connected. This can include a blood-pressure monitor, wireless or wired weight scale, wireless glucometer, wireless pulse oximeter, peak flow meter or stethoscope.

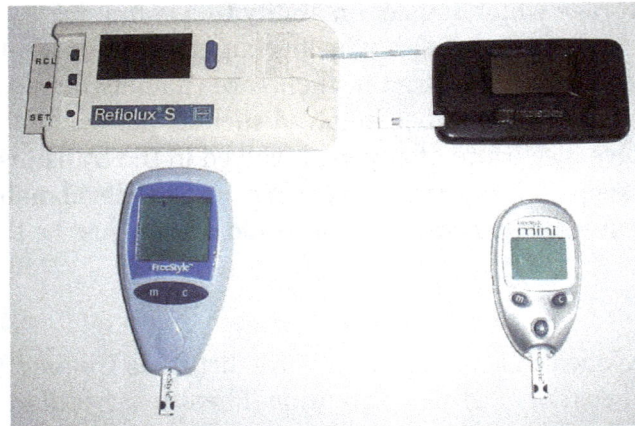

A THC unit can collect data on vital signs and health information from patients who entered values into the system. This is done manually or directly through the supplied peripherals. The data is transferred through telephone lines to a secure server located at the manufacturer's data centre. The data is then uploaded to a secure web-based application, allowing healthcare professionals to access and review patient information from any location with Internet access.

Applications

Based on research conducted in the United States by the Capital Area Consortium on Aging and Disability, the bandwidth of 128 Kbs was useful in a wide range of medical and nursing applications of THC. This includes:

- Patient interviews, histories, review of systems, activities of daily living;

- Follow-up assessment for functional mental status;

- Interventions not requiring physical presence;

- Supervision of physician assistants and nurse practitioners;

- Consultation with nursing colleagues and auxiliary services (physical therapy and occupational therapy);

- Medical consultations;

- Medication compliance;

- Patient education;

- Facilitation of case management;

- Triage in lieu of transport to emergency room or office; and

- Monitoring of vital signs, oximetry, electrocardiogram (ECG).

One of the applications of THC is providing nursing care using telephones, televisions, computers, and videoconferencing. THC can potentially improve patients outcomes, increase health care providers' productivity, and reduce health care costs. This application may be referred to as tele-nursing.

Cost-effectiveness

THC has demonstrated significant impact on hospital admissions and emergency room visits, as well as, walk-in clinic visits. Ontario Telemedicine Network (OTN) conducted a trial program that involved more than 800 patients with one of two chronic diseases - Congestive Heart Failure or COPD. The results were:

- 65% reduction in number of hospital admissions;

- 72% reduction in number of Emergency Room visits; and

- 95% reduction in number of walk-in clinic visits.

THC offers the opportunity to shift the delivery of many health care services from hospitals and other healthcare facilities to patients homes, thus reducing the load on the healthcare system and reserving hospitals for more critical cases. A recent study in The Journal of Telemedicine and Telecare, showed that very few studies have evaluated cost-effectiveness of THC, therefore, more research is needed to assess the value of THC in reducing costs associated with chronic disease management.

References

- Starfield, B.; Shi, L.; Macinko, J. (2005). "Contribution of primary care to health systems and health". The Milbank Quarterly. 83 (3): 457–502. doi:10.1111/j.1468-0009.2005.00409.x. PMC 2690145 . PMID 16202000

- Patient-Centered Primary Care Collaborative. "Joint Principles of the Patient Centered Medical Home". Retrieved 2 February 2012

- Wong, F.K.; Chung, L.C. (2006). "Establishing a definition for a nurse-led clinic: structure, process, and outcome". Journal of Advanced Nursing. 53 (3): 358–369. doi:10.1111/j.1365-2648.2006.03730.x. PMID 16441541

- Cooke, Brian (1990), The Grand Crimean Central Railway, Knutsford: Cavalier House, pp. 16–30, ISBN 0-9515889-0-7

- Hasted, Edward (1799). "Parishes". The History and Topographical Survey of the County of Kent. Institute of Historical Research. 6: 34–40. Retrieved 28 February 2014

- Ahmadi-Javid, A.; Seyedi, P.; Syam, S. (2017). "A Survey of Healthcare Facility Location". Computers & Operations Research. 79: 223–263. doi:10.1016/j.cor.2016.05.018

- Kaissi A, Shay P, Roscoe C. Hospital Systems, Convenient Care Strategies, and Healthcare Reform. Journal of Healthcare Management 61:2 March/April 2016

- Consultative Council on Medical and Allied Services (27 May 1920). "Interim Report on the Future Provision of Medical and Allied Services 1920 (Lord Dawson of Penn)". Socialist Health Association. Retrieved 21 December 2013

- Committee on the Future of Primary Care, Institute of Medicine (1996). Donaldson, Molla S.; Yordy, Karl D.; Lohr, Kathleen N.; Vanselow, Neal A., eds. Primary Care: America's Health in a New Era. Washington, DC: National Academies Press. ISBN 978-0-309-05399-0

- "Convention for the adaptation to maritime war of the principles of the Geneva Convention". Yale University. October 18, 1907. Retrieved August 2, 2009

- Sutherland Shaw, J.J. (1936). "The Hospital Ship, 1608–1740". The Mariner's Mirror. 22 (4): 422–426. doi:10 .1080/00253359.1936.10657206

- Corwin GS, Parker DM, Brown JR, Site of Treatment for Non-Urgent Conditions by Medicare Beneficiaries: Is there a role for Urgent Care Centres?, The American Journal of Medicine (2016), doi: 10.1016/j.amjmed.2016.03.013

- Webster, Charles (1998). The National Health Service A Political History. Oxford: Oxford University Press. p. 131. ISBN 0-19-289296-7

- "Statistical Communiqué on the 2011 National Economic and Social Development". stats.gov.cn. National Bureau of Statistics of China. 22 February 2012. Retrieved 2012-09-05

- Ershova I, Rider O, Gorelov V (December 2007). "Policlinics in London". Lancet. 370 (9603): 1890–1. doi:10.1016/S0140-6736(07)61793-0. PMID 18068500

- Fisher ES (September 2008). "Building a Medical Neighborhood for the Medical Home". The New England Journal of Medicine. 359 (12): 1202–5. doi:10.1056/NEJMp0806233. PMC 2729192 . PMID 18799556

- Bashshur, Rashid; Shannon, Gary William (2009-01-01). History of Telemedicine: Evolution, Context, and Transformation. Mary Ann Liebert. ISBN 9781934854112

- ""2012 Urgent Care Benchmarking Survey Results." Urgent Care Industry Information Kit. 2013" (PDF). Urgent Care Association of America. Retrieved 2015-06-26

- Wachter R, Goldman L (1996). "The emerging role of "hospitalists" in the American healthcare system". N Engl J Med. 335 (7): 514–7. doi:10.1056/NEJM199608153350713. PMID 8672160

- Wootton, R. (2012). Twenty years of telemedicine in chronic disease management – an evidence synthesis. In The Journal of Telemedicine and Telecare

- "Statistical Communiqué on the 2011 National Economic and Social Development". stats.gov.cn. National Bureau of Statistics of China. 2012-02-22. Archived from the original on August 6, 2012. Retrieved 2012-09-05

- Thobaben, M. (2005). Telehomecare. Home Health Care Management & Practice, 17(6), 487-488. doi: 10.1177/1084822305278125

- Maheu, Marlene; Whitten, Pamela; Allen, Ace (2002-02-28). E-Health, Telehealth, and Telemedicine: A Guide to Startup and Success. John Wiley & Sons. ISBN 9780787959036

- "H-160.919 Principles of the Patient-Centered Medical Home". American Medical Association Policy Finder. The American Medical Association. Retrieved 9 June 2014

- Wegner SE, Antonelli RC, Turchi RM (August 2009). "The medical home--improving quality of primary care for children" (PDF). Pediatr Clin North Am. 56 (4): 953–64. doi:10.1016/j.pcl.2009.05.021. PMID 19660637.

- Adamiak, E. Chojnacka, D. Walczak, Social security in Poland – cultural, historical and economical issues, Copernican Journal of Finance & Accounting, Vol 2, No 2, p. 23

3

A Brief Introduction to Health Care Management

Health administration is the management of hospitals, health care systems and public health systems. Hospital administrators may be generalists or specialists. Health care management is best understood in confluence with the major topics listed in the following section.

Health Administration

Health administration or healthcare administration is the field relating to leadership, management, and administration of public health systems, health care systems, hospitals, and hospital networks.

Terminology

Health systems management or health care systems management describes the leadership and general management of hospitals, hospital networks, and/or health care systems. In international use, the term refers to management at all levels. In the United States, management of a single institution (e.g. a hospital) is also referred to as "medical and health services management", "healthcare management", or "health administration".

Health systems management ensures that specific outcomes are attained, that departments within a health facility are running smoothly, that the right people are in the right jobs, that people know what is expected of them, that resources are used efficiently and that all departments are working towards a common goal.

Hospital Administrators

Hospital administrators are individuals or groups of people who act as the central point of control within hospitals. These individuals may be previous or current clinicians, or individuals with other backgrounds. There are two types of administrators, generalists and specialists. Generalists are individuals who are responsible for managing or helping to manage an entire facility. Specialists are individuals who are responsible for the efficient operations of a specific department such as policy analysis, finance, accounting, budgeting, human resources, or marketing.

It was reported in September 2014, that the United States spends roughly $218 billion per year on hospital's administration costs, which is equivalent to 1.43 percent of the total U.S. economy. Hospital administration has grown as a percent of the U.S. economy from .9 percent in 2000 to

1.43 percent in 2012, according to *Health Affairs*. In 11 different countries, hospitals allocate approximately 12 percent of their budget toward administrative costs. In the United States, hospitals spend 25 percent on administrative costs.

Competencies

NCHL competencies that require to engage with credibility, creativity, and motivation in complex and dynamic health care environments.

- Accountability
- Achievement orientation
- Change leadership
- Collaboration
- Communication skills
- Financial Skills
- Impact and influence
- Innovative thinking
- Organizational awareness
- Professionalism
- Self-confidence
- Strategic orientation
- Talent development
- Team leadership

Training and Organizations

Associated Qualifications

Health care management is usually studied through healthcare administration or healthcare management programs in a business school or, in some institutions, in a school of public health.

North America

Although many colleges and universities are offering a bachelor's degree in healthcare administration or human resources, a master's degree is considered the "standard credential" for most health administrators in the United States. Research and academic-based doctorate level degrees, such as the Doctor of Philosophy (PhD) in Health Administration and the Doctor of Health Administration (DHA) degree, prepare health care professionals to turn their clinical or administrative experiences into opportunities to develop new knowledge and practice, teach, shape public policy and/

or lead complex organizations. There are multiple recognized degree types that are considered equivalent from the perspective of professional preparation.

The Commission on the Accreditation of Healthcare Management Education (CAHME) is the accrediting body overseeing master's-level programs in the United States and Canada on behalf of the United States Department of Education. It accredits several degree program types, including Master of Hospital Administration (MHA), Master of Health Services Administration (MHSA), Master of Business Administration in Hospital Management (MBA-HM), Master of Health Administration (MHA), Master of Public Health (MPH, MSPH, MSHPM), Master of Science (MS-HSM, MS-HA), and Master of Public Administration (MPA).

Nepal

Health care management study is a new discipline in Nepal. Pokhara University offers a Hospital Management course. National Open College launched a four-year Bachelor's level (BHCM) course in September 2000 with an enrolment of 40 students, and the next year it also started a one-year postgraduate diploma (PGDHCM) and a two-year master's course (MHCM) in health care management. Nobel College at Sinamangal has also been offering a Bachelor's level (BHCM) course since 2006. MD Hospital administration (MDHA) and Master in Hospital Management (MHM) are being started from 2013. It is uncertain how many citizens of Nepal are gaining healthcare management qualifications in other countries. There is an absence of professional organization and regulation in the health care management profession in Nepal.

Professional Organizations

There are a variety of different professional associations related to health systems management, which can be subcategorized as either personal or institutional membership groups. Personal membership groups are joined by individuals, and typically have individual skills and career development as their focus. Larger personal membership groups include the American College of Healthcare Executives, the Healthcare Financial Management Association, and the Healthcare Information and Management Systems Society. Institutional membership groups are joined by organizations; whereas they typically focus on organizational effectiveness, and may also include data-sharing agreements and other medical related or administrative practice sharing vehicles for member organizations. Prominent examples include the American Hospital Association and the University Healthsystems Consortium.

History

Early hospital administrators were called patient directors or superintendents. At the time, many were nurses who had taken on administrative responsibilities. Over half of the members of the American Hospital Association were graduate nurses in 1916. Other superintendents were medical doctors, laymen and members of the clergy. In the United States, the first degree granting program in the United States was established at Marquette University in Milwaukee, Wisconsin. By 1927, the first two students received their degrees. The original idea is credited to Father Moulinier, associated with the Catholic Hospital Association. The first modern health systems management program was established in 1934 at the University of Chicago. At the time, programs were completed in two years – one year of formal graduate study and one year of practicing internship. In 1958, the Sloan program at Cornell University began offering a special program requiring two years of formal study, which remains the dominant structure in the United States and Canada today.

Health systems management has been described as a "hidden" health profession because of the relatively low-profile role managers take in health systems, in comparison to direct-care professions such as nursing and medicine. However the visibility of the management profession within healthcare has been rising in recent years, due largely to the widespread problems developed countries are having in balancing cost, access, and quality in their hospitals and health systems.

Operating Room Management

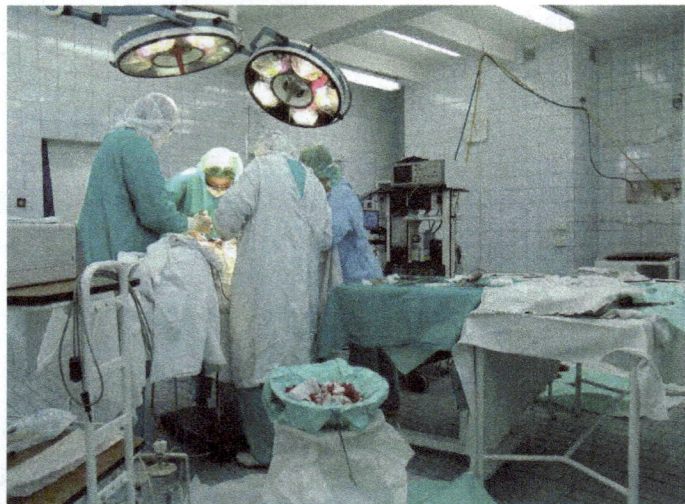

An operating theatre (gynecological hospital of Medical University of SilesiaBytom)

Operating room management is the science of how to run an Operating Room Suite. Operational operating room management focuses on maximizing operational efficiency at the facility, i.e. to maximize the number of surgical cases that can be done on a given day while minimizing the required resources and related costs. For example, what is the number of required anaesthetists or the scrub nurses that are needed next week to accommodate the expected workload or how can we minimize the cost of drugs used in the Operating Room? Strategic operating room management deals with long-term decision-making. For example, is it profitable to add two additional rooms to the existing facility? Typically, operating room management in profit-oriented health-care systems (e.g. United States) emphasizes strategic thinking whereas in countries with publicly funded health care (e.g. the UK), the focus is on operational decisions.

The act of coordinating and running all parts of a surgical suite to accomplish a defined set of goals. An emerging field, operating room management is increasingly studied as how to best: 1) ensure patient safety and optimal patient outcome, 2) provide surgeons with appropriate access to the OR so that patients can have operations in a timely manner, 3) maximize the efficiency of operating room utilization, staff, and materials, 4) decrease patient delays, 5) enhance satisfaction among patients, staff, and physicians.

This management science as applied to the surgical suite is gaining more attention because of increasing market pressures on hospitals from competitors (e.g., other surgical suites including office based surgery) and from payers seeking lower prices. The surgical suite is often considered a profitable hospital unit. As such, surgical suites also comprise an important fraction of hospital budget spending. Holding patient safety constant, the opportunity to increase financial gain through modifying the use of already existing resources is a prime target for managerial analysis. Incremental improvements in operating room utilization and operating room efficiency can have major impacts on hospital staff and finances. Some hospital administrators perceive efficiency in the operating room as throughput, completing the most surgical cases within budget.

Surgical Suite Personnel

The management of a surgical suite must take into account all cooperating team members. The operating environment consists of interaction between surgeons, anesthesiologists, nurses, technicians, and patients.

The Necessity of Management

Overhead costs include, but are not limited to, the space, technology and devices, pharmaceuticals and staffing. Hospital administrators have consequently focused their attention towards maximizing OR profitability, and thereby hospital profitability, through contribution margins. This focus, in addition to the boom in demand for elective surgery, has led to a rapid growth of OR facilities. Historically, nurses have been chiefly responsible for the daily functioning of the surgical suite. Increasingly, facilities are hiring a physician medical director for the OR, as represented by a surgeon, anesthesiologist, or both. In some instances, all three branches of surgery, anesthesia, and nursing will be represented in the daily OR management infrastructure. By working collegially, these three fields can mobilize all resources necessary to maximize OR productivity. Because medical needs and regulatory requirements are constantly changing, the concept of appointing a medical director in the OR, an operating room manager, has gained acceptance.

Clinicians typically focus on operational decisions on the day of surgery (short term) such as moving cases from one OR to another, assigning and relieving staff, prioritizing urgent cases, and scheduling add-on case. On the other hand, upper management typically focuses on strategic decision making (long term) such as whether to open a new cancer center, or whether to align the hospital with a regional health care system.

Principles of Operating Room Management

The decisions made by OR management should have a clear and definitive purpose in order to maintain consistency. In order of priority, governing principles of OR managers are to: (1) ensure patient safety and the highest quality of care; (2) provide surgeons with appropriate access to the OR; (3) maximize the efficiency of operating room utilization, staff, and materials to reduce costs; (4) decrease patient delays; and (5) enhance satisfaction among patients, staff, and physicians. If OR management is properly performed ahead of time, all that doctors and nurses have to think about on the day of surgery is the patient. If management is poor, then the medical and nursing staff may waste efforts and resources to rush cases or juggle schedules, thus compromising attention to patient safety.

Operating Room Utilization

OR utilization is a measure of the use of an operating room that is properly staffed with people needed to successfully deliver a surgical procedure to a patient.

Block Utilization is a measure of the use of operating room time by a surgeon or group of surgeons to whom time has been allocated.

Raw utilization is the total hours of elective cases performed within OR time divided by the hours of allocated block time.

Raw Utilization = total hours of cases performed ÷ total hours of OR time allocated

Adjusted utilization uses the total hours of elective cases performed within OR block time, including "credit" for the turnover times necessary to set up and clean up ORs.

Adjusted Utilization = [total hours of cases + "credit time"] ÷ total hours of OR time allocated

Factors affecting utilization rates include: the accuracy of estimated case times, cancellation rate, number of add-ons available to fill gaps, longest cases go first, the time of day as utilization typically is highest in the morning and lowest in the evening, outpatient centers have lower utilization, and other constraints (i.e., surgeon can only use room 12, or start at 11 am).

Improvements in operating room efficiency can have a major impact on hospital staff and finances as well as operating room management.

Operating Room Efficiency

Operating room (OR) efficiency is a measure of how well time and resources are used for their intended purposes. One way to analyze efficiency is to chart *under-utilized* and *over-utilized* time spent on a given day in the operating room. If the cases in an operating room finish earlier than scheduled, time is *under-utilized*. Likewise, if the cases in an operating room run "late" or past its allotted operating room time then this produces *over-utilized time*.

The terms *operating room utilization* and *operating room productivity* are also often used when discussing operating room management of a surgical suite.

Performance Dashboard for a Surgical Suite

An operating room manager must select criteria, key performance indicators, or a dashboard of measurements, to assess overall functioning of a surgical suite. An example of an analytic tool used to rate surgical suites is reflected below. This scoring system was created in order to quantify the efficiency levels of surgical suites. Its economical efficacy has yet to be validated by formal studies. In addition, it was developed in the US and contains scoring elements that are applicable for an American surgical suite. It is therefore unlikely to be useful for operating room managers outside the US.

OR efficiency measurements

Measurements	poor performance	medium performance	high performance
Excess Staffing Costs	>10%	5-10%	<5%
Start-time tardiness (mean tardiness for elective cases/day)	>60 min	45-60 min	<45 min
Case cancellation rate	>10%	5-10%	<5%
Post Anesthesia Care Unit (PACU) admission delays (% workdays with at least one delay in PACU admission)	>20%	10-20%	<10%
Contribution Margin (mean) per operating room hour	<$1,000/hr	$1–2,000/hr	>$2,000/hr
Turnover Time (for all cases mean time from previous patient out of the OR to next patient in the OR including set-up and cleanup)	>40 min	25-40 min	<25 min
Prediction Bias (bias in case duration estimates per 8 hours of operating room time)	>15 min	5-15 min	<5 min
Prolonged turnovers (% turnovers lasting more than 60 minutes)	>25%	10-25%	<10%

The above objective criteria can be computed from data commonly available in hospital administrative data systems.

Excess Staffing Costs

Nothing is more important than to first allocate the right amount of OR time to each service on each day of the week for their case scheduling. This is not the same as the block time! To illustrate this imagine that two cases each lasting 2 hours are scheduled into OR #1 with OR nurses and an anesthesiologist scheduled to work an 8 hr day. The matching of workload to staffing has been so poor that little can be done the day of surgery to increase the efficiency of use of the staff. Neither awakening patients more quickly nor reducing the turnover time, for example, will compensate for the poor initial choice of staffing for OR #1 and/or how the cases were scheduled into OR #1.

Optimal allocation of OR time should be based on historical use by a particular service (i.e., unit of OR allocation such as surgeon, group, department, or specialty) and then using computer software to minimize the amount of underutilized time and the more expensive overutilized time. Under-utilized hours reflect how early the room finishes. In the example above, if staff were scheduled to work from 7:00 am to 3:00 pm and instead the room finished at 11 am, then there would be 4 hours of underutilized time. The excess staffing cost would be 50% (4 hours/8 hours). On the other hand, if 9 hours of cases are performed in an OR with staff scheduled to work 8 hours then the excess staffing cost is 25%. Over-utilized hours are the hours that ORs run longer than the regularly scheduled OR hours, or 1 hr in this example. 1hr/8hr=12.5% which is then multiplied by the additional cost of staying late, which often is assumed to be a factor of two (related to monetary overtime cost paid to staff, as well as recruitment and retention costs related to unhappy staff because they have to stay late unpredictably). OR suites can reasonably aim to achieve a staffing cost that is within 10% of optimal (i.e., workload is perfectly matched to staffing).

If the key is to allocate appropriate time to each service based on historical OR use, how do you deal with rooms consistently running late on the day of surgery? The answer: make the allocated time, into which cases are being scheduled, longer. For example, if a surgeon does 12 hours worth of cases every day he is in the OR, don't plan 8 hours of staffing (7am-3pm) and have everyone frustrated by having to stay late (overtime). Rather, schedule his cases into 12 hours of allocated time (7am-7pm). That way, anesthesia and nursing staff know they will be there 12 hours when they arrive to work and overtime costs (financial and morale) will be reduced. The common response to this approach is, "No one wants to be there till 7 pm." The answer to that is, "You are there now till 7 pm so why not make scheduled OR time 12 hr long and have a more predictable work day duration." Thus, optimizing staffing costs is finding balance between overtime and finishing early.

There may be concern about a nurse manager's ability to flex the staff enough to avoid excess staffing costs. It can be difficult from a human resources standpoint to match scheduled cases with staffing perfectly, such that staff still get the hours and shifts they need. For example, if Dr Smith needs a 12-hour block, the manager needs to find staff who want to work a 12-hour shift (or part-timers in some combination). Staffing is not only an OR efficiency issue, but a staff satisfaction issue. It can be a challenge at a time when recruiting and retaining nurses are growing concerns.

Start-time Tardiness

Start-time tardiness is the mean tardiness of start times for elective cases per OR per day. Reducing the time patients have to wait for their surgery once they arrive to the hospital (especially if the preceding case runs late) is another important goal for the OR manager. If a case is supposed to start at 10:00 am (patient enters OR), but the case starts at 10:30 am instead, then there are 30 minutes of tardiness. In computing this metric, no credit is given if the 10:00 am case starts early (for example at 9:45 am).

The tardiness of start of scheduled cases should total less than 45 mins per eight-hour OR day in well functioning OR suites. Facilities with long work days will have greater tardiness because the longer the day, the more uncertainty about case start times. Having patients' medical records ready to go with all needed documents is essential for on time starts.

Case Cancellation Rate on Day of Surgery

Cancellation rates vary among facilities, depending partly on the types of patients receiving care, ranging from 4.6% for outpatients, to 13% -18% at VA medical centers. Many cancellations are due to non-medical problems such as a full ICU, surgeon unavailability, or bad weather. OR cancellation rates can be monitored statistically. Well functioning OR suites should have cancellation rates less than 5%. Monitoring the cancellations correctly is calculated by taking the ratio of the number of cancellations to the number of scheduled cases.

PACU Admission Delays

PACU admission delays can be expressed as a % of workdays with at least one delay of 10 mins or greater in PACU admission because PACU is full. It is important to adjust PACU nurse staffing around the times of OR admissions. Algorithms exist that use the number of available nursing hours to find the staffing solution with the fewest number of understaffed days.

Contribution Margin Per OR Hour

An OR suite that puts up with excessive surgical times can schedule itself efficiently but still lose its financial shirt if many surgeons are slow, use too many instruments, or expensive implants, etc.

These are all measured by the contribution margin per OR hr. The contribution margin per hour of OR time is the hospital revenue generated by a surgical case, less all the hospitalization variable labor and supply costs. Variable costs, such as implants, vary directly with the volume of cases performed.

This is because fee-for-service hospitals have a positive contribution margin for almost all elective cases mostly due to a large percentage of OR costs being fixed. For USA hospitals not on a fixed annual budget, contribution margin per OR hour averages one to two thousand USD per OR hour.

Turnover Times

Turnover time is the time from when one patient exits an OR until the next patient enters the same OR. Turnover times include cleanup times and setup times, but not delays between cases. Based on data collected at 31 USA hospitals, turnover times at the best performing OR suites average less than 25 mins. Cost reduction from reducing turnover times (because OR workload is less) can only be achieved if OR allocations and staffing are reduced. Despite this, turnover time receives lots of attention from OR managers because it is a key satisfier for surgeons.

Sometimes the OR suite reduces turnover times (by providing more staff to clean the room for example) but new problems arise (not enough time for sterilizing instruments for the new case, can't bring patient to PACU because no beds) that were "hidden" by long turnover times.

Times between cases that are longer than a defined interval (e.g., 1 hr because to follow surgeon is unavailable) should be considered delays, not turnovers.

Prediction Bias

Prediction bias in case duration are expressed as estimates per 8 hr of OR time. Prediction error equals the actual duration of the new case minus the estimated duration of the new case. Bias indicates whether the estimate is consistently too high or consistently too low, and precision reflects the magnitudes of the errors of the estimates. Efficient OR suites should aim to have bias in case duration estimates per 8 hr of OR time that is less than 15 minutes. A reason for bias can be surgeons' consistently shortening their case duration estimates because they have too little OR time allocated and need to "fit" their list of cases into the OR time they do have. In contrast, other OR suites may have surgeons that purposely overestimate case durations to keep control/access of their allocated OR time so that if a new case appears their OR time was not given away.

Remember that lack of historical case duration data for scheduled procedures is an important cause of inaccuracy in predicting case duration. In general, half of the cases scheduled in your OR suite tomorrow will have less than five previous cases of the same procedure type and same surgeon during the preceding year.

It would be nice to have no uncertainty in case duration prediction. But, it is present. The problem is looking for a single number that is correct most of the time. You won't get accurate estimates by using historical case duration data. Rather, from the historical data you'll get an assessment of the uncertainty.

Prolonged Turnovers

Times between cases that are longer than a defined interval. (note: late arrival of a surgeon should be considered delays, not turnovers.)

Operating Room Productivity

Operating room productivity is the quantity and quality of output (typically surgical cases) from the surgical suite in contrast to the amount of input required (such as physicians and nurses and equipment for example). Many institutions believe that productivity (output/input) can be accomplished without sacrificing convenience (rapid access to open OR time such that a surgeon can book a case without having to wait) but these two aspects are not separable.

Typically, the greater the *operating room utilization*, the less the convenience (able to book cases when desired) as defined by surgeons and patients. This is because as utilization goes up there is less available open staffed OR time available on short notice. In other words, the greater the access and convenience, the lower is *operating room utilization* (because of the need for extra capacity), at least as perceived by hospitals and anesthesiologists. This high level of customer service of being able to book cases on short notice is one reason ambulatory surgery centers typically have lower OR utilization than big city hospitals. The outpatient surgery center usually has reduced overhead when compared to a big city hospital, and therefore can financially get away with lower OR use.

Sociopolitical Factors in Management of the Surgery Suite: *"OR Equilibrium"*

Management of the operating room suite must acknowledge that people are the primary resource. Although management science theory may tend to hold constant the preferences and bias of the individuals working in and utilizing the surgery suite, management of the surgical suite with regards to case scheduling is strongly influenced by personal, political, and economic relationships within an institution.

Who is the Main Customer of your Surgical Suite?

To best align management goals with institutional objectives the OR director needs to identify the primary customer of the surgical suite. An OR can be completely balanced or it can be biased to one or more its constituents. The main people to consider are surgeons, anesthesiologists, nurses, the hospital (upper management), and of course the patient.

A first step is to determine whose preferences or workload dominates the surgical suite. If surgeons are in large demand with small supply, then that may outweigh other interests. For example, a private facility may have surgeons who can pull their patients to another hospital if made to wait. As another example, in a private surgeon-owned surgery center, management may be directed as maintaining a particular partner's workload and the incentives are to schedule his/her cases with priority.

The same supply/demand balance applies to anesthesia. The situation may exist where a specific surgery group will only work with its contracted anesthesia group. In this case, a manager may have to wait until the contracted anesthesiologist is ready for the case, even if this means idle OR time. This can be avoided in institutions where one group has exclusive rights and controls anesthesia privilege over all the ORs. This arrangement is seen commonly because it eliminates factions and streamlines anesthesia placement for cases, either elective or emergency.

Hospital (Upper Management) run ORs are identified by those facilities where the hospital executives acting as agents for government authorities determine staffing and workload. Examples include hospitals in public health care systems like in European countries or the VA United States Department of Veteran Affairs in the USA.

In other surgical suites, in contrast, management decisions have patients as the first priority. Facilities performing elective cosmetic procedures for cash reimbursement are an example. Due to the patient being able to choose where they have plastic surgery, patients expect special circumstances such as first-rate customer service. Additionally, if a patient is one hour late for surgery the patient will most likely still be able to undergo surgery. This concept is in contrast to a large academic hospital, for example, where a patient who misses their check-in window for elective surgery is often removed from the surgery schedule to make room for re-shuffled elective and emergency cases.

What are the Preferences of the Main Customer in the Surgical Suite?

Once the manager has identified the critical few customers and the necessary many customers, then the next step is to determine their preferences and incentives. Surgeons will favor early block surgery times, rapid turnover, low cancellation rates, and on time starts. The hospital (upper management) will want the most surgical output with the least associated cost. Patients will likely favor reduced waiting times for surgery start. Finally, nurse managers and anesthesiologists will be inclined to high operating room utilization, minimal overtime, the flexibility to move cases around, and reserve capacity in the ORs.

Much like economic Game Theory, agents in the OR will position their interests in a nature as to maximize their returns. It is up to the OR manager to weigh the contributions of each agent and provide enough OR time and resources to maximize the output of the surgical suite in its entirety.

Theory and Applications of Operating Room Management

This discussion addresses capitalistic healthcare markets. A discussion of socialized medicine would include several other factors which influence the supply and demand for surgical care. Analysis of operating room management within socialized medicine is becoming increasingly frequent in the medical literature.

A manager must select benchmarks in order to analyze changes from baseline operations. Upgrades to existing operating infrastructures should be demonstrated as efficiency gained compared to baseline practices. Management criteria must therefore include preoperative, intraoperative, and immediate postoperative system analysis.

Preoperative Management Issues

Waiting time and *operating room scheduling* are the two key preoperative determinates.

Waiting time prior to operation The time from surgical scheduling to check-in for the procedure is defined, for these purposes, as "preoperative wait time."

Use of a surgical suite depends greatly on, and increases as, the average length of time patients wait for surgery increases. As waiting time increases, more surgical dates (blocks) can be evaluated for a good match between a case's duration and the open times in the blocks. In some communities, competition among surgeons and hospitals may not allow the average length of time that patients have to wait for surgery to be as long as 2 weeks. An OR suite then cannot expect block time utilization from elective cases to exceed 90%, assuming that enough block time is allocated for a surgeon to complete all of the elective cases in the block time.

For these purposes, wait time can be equated to the price of an object. The price for an object increases if demand increases and/or supply reduces for that object. Hence, "preoperative wait time" will increase as demand for surgery increases and/or surgical supply (operating room availability) reduces or fails to grow proportionally to surgical demand.

By accurately gauging a patient population and an operative facility's capacity, an effective manager can minimize the wait for elective and imminent procedures while covering all emergency cases and without overextending the operative team.

Scheduling Operating Room Calendars

Case scheduling or correctly selecting the day on which to do each elective case so as to best fill the allocated hours is most important, much more so than, for example, correcting errors in predicting how long elective or add-on cases would last, reducing variability in turnover or delays between cases, or day-to-day variation in hours of add-on cases.

Poor scheduling is often the cause of lost OR time. To more efficiently operate a surgical setting, managers may consider centralizing all scheduling to the operating room suite itself. Ideally, holding patient and surgeon preferences constant, an operating facility can identify cases and appropriately place them into predetermined time slots, or blocks.

To examine scheduling challenges, consider three possible surgical scenarios: elective (e.g. cosmetic procedures, stable situations not increasing in severity), imminent (e.g. inflamed gall bladder removal, potential for worsening harm if situations not surgically corrected,) and emergency surgeries (e.g. burst appendix, situations in which death or disability is possible or likely). The majority of operative time is a combination of elective and imminent surgeries. Albeit a smaller percentage, emergency surgical cases must always be handled promptly in order to ensure patient safety. Emergency surgeries are often unforeseeable and present a scheduling challenge as a result. Therefore, from a management perspective, one must use the elective and imminent surgical cases as a guideline for pre-determining operative schedules, while allowing flexibility for the emergency situations that indubitably arise.

The historical approach for scheduling operating room time is via analysis of previous surgical information. For example, to estimate how much time a cholecystectomy will require, the management determines how long previous cholecystectomy operations took the participating surgeon. Limiting this approach is the number of prior recorded cases and the surgeon's familiarity with the procedure. Previously recorded information serves to set a precedent for turnover rates. By allowing surgeons to operate efficiently based on their previous timetables, a manager allows all parties involved to work more efficiently.

Nothing is more important than to first allocate the right amount of OR time to each service on each day of the week so that rarely do services fill their allocated OR time and have another case to schedule. This allocation is based on historical use by surgeon and then using computer to minimize ratio of underutilized time and over-utilized time (which is more expensive).

A prevailing school of thought is for managers to allocate operating room time based on the principles of safety, access and operating room efficiency, in respective order of importance. Part of a manager's job is to clearly communicate these factors to all parties involved in care delivery.

There are times when a departmental manager must realize a departure from this practice and intervene to save profitability margins. For instance, an anesthesia practice group may negotiate extra funds from their employer (university, hospital, multi-specialty medical groups) to compensate for underutilized operating room time. In this instance, an anesthesia manager may use predetermined formulas to estimate excess labor costs they incur that are not offset by proper operating room utilization. A manager, whether departmental of administrative, that uses proactive applications can eliminate inefficiencies within their operating systems.

Intraoperative Management Issues

Managers need to evaluate: 1) operating room leadership; 2) departmental leadership within the operating room; 3) interpersonal conflicts amongst the operating team; 4) physical layout and location of the operating room in relation to other integral departments; 5) operating room communication systems; and 6) patient turnover.

Only then can options such as providing rewards and incentives for improved operating room efficiency, assessing logistical and system design, delegating responsibility, and implementing teamwork initiatives be instituted to produce more favorable outcomes for both the provider and the patient.

Surgical Suite Leadership

Generally, an institution or private surgery center will have an agreed upon leader, generally dubbed the "Operating Room Manager." The reporting structure is typically to a VP of surgical services. A manager may have the business and academic ability to operate a facility, but without the cooperation of staff and practitioners, most reform efforts will be futile.

An OR manager must be in compliance with several internal and external governing bodies. Depending on the institution, a given manager may have to work closely with committees ranging from patient safety and medical staff safety boards to an auxiliary OR committee. The Joint Commission on Accreditation of Healthcare Organizations (JCAHO) and the Centers for Medicare and Medicaid Services (CMS) puts forth an external, universal regulatory standard for hospitals and ORs. An OR manager must maintain compliance with this spectrum of policies in order to maintain both patient safety as well as hospital accreditation. One of many notable policies put forth by JHACO [Joint Commission] is the universal protocol, implemented to ensure patient safety. This protocol requires that three sequential events must be completed prior to surgical incision in order to reduce iatrogenic errors and postoperative complications. The three checkpoints are (1) preoperative verification of procedure and background information, (2) marking of the operative site with a marker and surgeon's initials, and (3) an official timeout for an audible confirmation of patient identity and the procedure to be completed. These regulations have proven to reduce avoidable complications of intraoperative mistakes and resultant postoperative morbidities and mortalities.

Departmental Leadership within the Surgical Suite

This topic compartmentalizes each member of a surgical suite team to his/her department (e.g. surgery, anesthesiology, environmental services, housekeeping, etc.). The principle behind departmental leadership is the delegation of responsibility. An operating room manager must rely upon departments to uphold their respective regulations in addition to acting in the best interest of the overall institution. This interest directly relates to operating room utilization and operating room productivity. Therefore, a surgical chief must be an active member of scheduling block time for surgery in order to avoid persistent over or underutilization of resources.

Interpersonal Conflicts Amongst the Surgical Suite Team

The majority of accidents in technical professions have human error as causal elements. More critically, these errors tend to involve interpersonal issues: communications, leadership, conflict, flawed decision making, etc. A questionnaire circulated to operating room staff and professionals identified communication problems as an overwhelming barrier to operating room performance. This problem is a constant theme within healthcare and can disrupt an operating room and detract from operating room efficiency. It is imperative that a manager optimize personal issues and act quickly to correct them.

Physical Layout and Location of the Surgical Suite in Relation to Other Integral Departments (i.e. Radiology, Pathology, etc.)

An effective manager must analyze the layout of each operating room individually and as a whole. The mass of new technologies and equipment, such as Endoscopic surgical procedures, in today's operating room is increasing. Crowding may adversely affect the abilities of the surgical team. Managers must act to appropriately modify pre-existing operating room space or by identifying key design issues during the conception and building of new facilities. Larger cases where more materials and instruments are used should be appropriately scheduled into rooms that can accommodate them.

Likewise, the surgical suite ideally is placed in close proximity to support functions such as radiology, pathology, and intensive care. Creating unnecessary distance between these entities compromises both operating room efficiency and patient safety.

Surgical Suite Communication Systems and Patient Turnover

Current technologies provide managers with tools to reduce patient turnover rate. Standard practices include passive status displays (whiteboards or screens in the surgical suites) and active displays (text pager notifications). These communication tools streamline interdisciplinary planning for real time decision-making. A recent study suggests going further and implementing a system of command displays (text suggestions of how to act) or even patient tracking systems such as with RFID tags. This communication is essential to know when to expect patients to arrive to the holding area prior to entering the OR, or to the recovery room after surgery.

Reduction in turnover time (patient exists operating room until next patient enters operating room) requires all individuals in the surgical suite to work together. The day-to-day management of operating room efficiency is integral to the maximization of both qualitative (improved professional satisfaction) and quantitative (completion of more cases and reduced staffing costs) returns.

Postoperative Operating Room Management

Surgical Care Improvement Project (SCIP)

SCIP is a national partnership of organizations that are dedicated to reducing postoperative complications.

The project focuses on four broad areas in which the incidence and cost of complications are high: (1) Surgical site infections, (2) Perioperative myocardial infarctions (heart attacks), (3) Venous thromboembolism, and (4) Postoperative pneumonia.

An operating room manager must consider the preoperative, intraoperative and postoperative factors which reflect in patient safety and hospital efficiency. Ideally, a manager is approachable, intelligent, and an effective leader who communicates well with hospital staff. The above techniques and principles highlight many of the ways in which a manager can successfully direct a surgical suite to maximize its benefit to the patients, staff and hospital

Bed Management

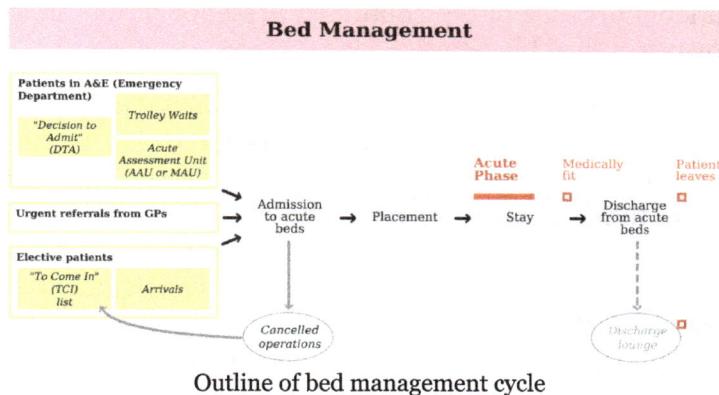

Outline of bed management cycle

Bed management is the allocation and provision of beds, especially in a hospital where beds in specialist wards are a scarce resource. The "bed" in this context represents not simply a place for the patient to sleep, but the services that go with being cared for by the medical facility: admission processing, physician time, nursing care, necessary diagnostic work, appropriate treatment, and so forth.

In the UK, acute hospital bed management is usually performed by a dedicated team and may form part of a larger process of patient flow management.

Importance

Because hospital beds are economically scarce resources, there is naturally pressure to ensure high occupancy rates and therefore a minimal buffer of empty beds. However, because the volume of emergency admissions is unpredictable, hospitals with average occupancy levels above 85 per cent "can expect to have regular bed shortages and periodic bed crises."

Shortage of beds can result in cancellations of admissions for planned (elective) surgery, admission to inappropriate wards (medical vs. surgical, male vs. female etc.), delay admitting emergency patients, and transfers of existing inpatients between wards, which "will add a day to a patient's length of stay".

These can be politically sensitive issues in publicly funded healthcare systems. In the UK there has been concern over inaccurate and sometimes fraudulently manipulated waiting list statistics, and claims that "the current A&E target is simply not achievable without the employment of dubious management tactics." In 2013 two Stafford Hospital nurses were struck off the nursing register for falsifying A&E discharge times between 2000 and 2010 to avoid breaches of four-hour waiting targets.

Specific Problems

- *Shortage of beds due to lack of other options.* Hospitals in developed countries cannot force a patient to leave if the patient's home is reasonably believed to be unsafe. For example, if a frail, elderly patient has recovered from an acute illness, but is unable to dress himself and prepare simple meals on his own, then the hospital must ensure that the patient will have sufficient assistance with these necessary activities of daily living, or the patient must remain in the hospital. In places with a shortage of skilled nursing facilities, home health care workers, and related support organizations, beds may be unavailable for new, acutely sick patients because of the continued presence of the previous patients. This is sometimes known as a "bed blocking".

- *False appearance or unnecessary creation of a bed shortage.* "Bed hiding", as it is sometimes called, is the practice of delaying admissions due to a falsely claimed lack of beds in the appropriate department. Bed hiding has several causes, including scheduling so many elective procedures that there are inadequate beds left for emergency admissions; frequent changes from ward to ward; inadequate communication, so that cleaning staff don't know when a bed has become available and needs cleaning; misalignment of tasks, so that skilled nurses are expected to take time away from direct patient care to clean beds; too few nurses scheduled for a shift; and overworked staff, who may be inclined to mis-report a bed as full, especially at the end of a shift, in an effort to shift the workload to another person. Bed hiding can be significantly reduced by careful tracking of bed status, making cleaning after discharge the top priority for cleaning staff, and even by physically moving patients to the ward as soon as they are ready for admission rather than boarding them in the emergency department. Reducing bed hiding in regular wards can reduce wait times in the emergency department.

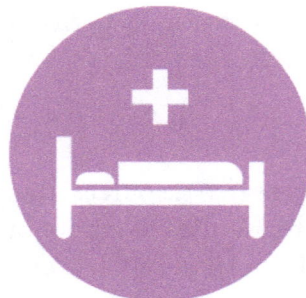

Health Information Management

Health information management (HIM) is information management applied to health and health care. It is the practice of acquiring, analyzing and protecting digital and traditional medical information vital to providing quality patient care. With the widespread computerization of health records, traditional (paper-based) records are being replaced with electronic health records (EHRs). The tools of health informatics and health information technology are continually improving to bring greater efficiency to information management in the health care sector. Both hospital information systems and health human resources information systems (HRHIS) are common implementations of HIM.

Health information management professionals plan information systems, develop health policy, and identify current and future information needs. In addition, they may apply the science of informatics to the collection, storage, analysis, use, and transmission of information to meet legal, professional, ethical and administrative records-keeping requirements of health care delivery. They work with clinical, epidemiological, demographic, financial, reference, and coded healthcare data. Health information administrators have been described to "play a critical role in the delivery of healthcare in the United States through their focus on the collection, maintenance and use of quality data to support the information-intensive and information-reliant healthcare system".

The World Health Organization (WHO) stated that the proper collection, management and use of information within healthcare systems "will determine the system's effectiveness in detecting health problems, defining priorities, identifying innovative solutions and allocating resources to improve health outcomes".

History and Development of HIM Standards in the United States

HIM Standards Began with Establishment of AHIMA

Health information management's standards history is dated back to the introduction of the American Health Information Management Association, founded in 1928 "when the American College of Surgeons established the Association of Record Librarians of North America (ARLNA) to 'elevate the standards of clinical records in hospitals and other medical institutions.'"

In 1938, AHIMA was known as American Association of Medical Record Librarians (AAMRL) and its members were known as medical record experts or librarians who studied medical record science. The goal was to raise the standards of records keeping in hospitals and other healthcare facilities. The individuals involved in this profession were promoters for the successful management of clinical records to guarantee accuracy and precision. Over time, the organization's name changed to reflect the evolving field of health information management practices, eventually becoming the American Health Information Management Association. The association's current name is meant to cover the wide variety of areas which health professionals work in today.

AHIMA members affect the quality of patient information and patient care at every touch point in the healthcare delivery cycle. They often serve in bridge roles, connecting clinical, operational, and administrative functions.

HIMSs Establishment in 1961 Increased Industry Knowledge

The Healthcare Information and Management Systems Society (HIMSS) was organized in 1961 as the Hospital Management Systems Society (HMSS), an independent, unincorporated, nonprofit, voluntary association of individuals. It was preceded by increasing amounts of management engineering activity in healthcare during the 1950s, when teachings of Frederick Winslow Taylor and Frank Bunker Gilbreth, Sr. began to attract the attention of health leaders.

The HIMSS grew to include chapters, membership categories, publications, conventions, and continues to grow in different parts of the world via its Europe, Asia Pacific, and Middle Eastern branches.

Accredited HIM Educational Program Development

The Commission on Accreditation for Health Informatics and Information Management Education (CAHIIM) defines standards which higher education health information management and technology programs must meet to qualify for accreditation. Students who graduate from an accredited associate's, bachelor's or certificate program are qualified to sit for their respective exams for certification as a Registered Health Information Technician (RHIT) – via graduation from an accredited associate or certification program or Registered Health Information Administrator (RHIA), which requires education through an accredited bachelor or certification program. Competency requirements are maintained by CAHIIM in their Associate Degree Entry-Level Competencies and Baccalaureate Degree Entry-Level Competencies definitions.

Modern Development

Electronic Health Records

The electronic health record has been continually expressed as an evolvement of health record-keeping. Because it is electronic, this means of record keeping has been both supported and debated in the health professional community and within the public realm.

In the United States, 89% of those who responded to a recent Wall Street Journal poll described themselves as "Very/Somewhat Confident" in their health care provider who used electronic health records compared to 71% of respondents who responded positively about their providers who didn't or don't use electronic health records. As of 2008, more than fifty-percent of Chief Information Officers polled listed that they wanted ambulatory electronic health records in order to have the health information record available to move across each stage of health care.

Health information managers are charged with the protection of patient privacy and are responsible for training their employees in the proper handling and usage of the confidential information entrusted to them. With the rise of technology's importance in healthcare, health information managers must remain competent with the use of information databases that generate crucial reports for administrators and physicians.

Educational Programs

The requisites and accreditation processes for health information management education and professional activity vary across jurisdictions.

In the United States, the CAHIIM requires continued accreditation for accredited programs in health information management. The current standard is that accreditation may be maintained with periodic site visits, submission of an annual report, informing CAHIIM of adverse changes within the program and paying CAHIIM administrative fees. HIM students may opt to participate in a full-time bridge program called the Joint Bachelor of Science/Masters Program. With this program, students can achieve both the Bachelor of Science in Health Information Management and the Master of Health Services Administration Program (BSHIM/MHSA). The full-time bridge program allows students to achieve both degrees in five years. Students pursuing the BSHIM/ MHSA will be prepared to assume management and executive positions in health-related organizations such as: hospitals, managed care organizations, health information system developers and vendors, and pharmaceutical companies, and bring their knowledge in HIM to these positions.

In Canada, graduates of Canadian Health Information Management Association (CHIMA) programs are eligible to write a national certification examination to pursue a profession in HIM.

Online Program Availability

There are many programs that are also available online. Online students collaborate with in-class students using internet technology. With online learning, students are allowed to go through the programs at their own pace. Online students are included in class through group lectures that are recorded and put online, discussion boards and are members of group projects with in-class students. Some online students are even allowed to attend some classes on campus and take some classes online.

Further Education for Health Information Professionals

Education is an important aspect in being successful in the world of health information management. Aside from initial credentials, health information professionals may wish to pursue a Masters of Health Information Management, Masters of Business Administration, Masters of Health Administration, or other Masters programs in health data management, information technology and systems, and organization and management. Gaining further education advances the health professional's career and qualifies the individual for upper-management positions.

Canada (CHIMA)

In Canada, current HIM employees are mostly called the "Health Information Management Professionals", with the designation of "Certified Health Information Manager" (CHIM). The accrediting association here is the Canadian Health Information Management Association (CHIMA). The following list below consists of Canadian post-secondary schools that have given full accreditation for their HIM programs from CHIMA:

Diploma Level

- Alberta: Southern Alberta Institute of Technology in Calgary
- British Columbia: Douglas College in Coquitlam

- Manitoba: Red River College in Winnipeg
- New Brunswick: New Brunswick Community College in Moncton
- Nova Scotia: Nova Scotia Community College in Halifax
- Ontario: Fleming College in Peterborough
- Ontario: George Brown College in Toronto
- Ontario: St. Lawrence College in Kingston
- Ontario: Westervelt College in London
- Quebec: Collège Laflèche in Trois-Rivières
- Quebec: O'Sullivan College in Montreal
- Saskatchewan: Saskatchewan Polytechnic in Regina

Bachelor Degree Level

- Ontario: Conestoga College in Kitchener
- Ontario: Ryerson University in Toronto

Distance Learning

- Nova Scotia: Heritage Professional Centre in Sydney
- Ontario: HealthCareCAN/CHA Learning in Ottawa
- Saskatchewan: Saskatchewan Polytechnic in Regina

Elements

Healthcare quality and safety require that the right information be available at the right time to support patient care and health system management decisions. Gaining consensus on essential data content and documentation standards is a necessary prerequisite for high-quality data in the interconnected healthcare system of the future. Continuous quality management of data standards and content is key to ensuring that information is usable and actionable.

Records

- The patient health record is the primary legal record documenting the health care services provided to a person in any aspect of the health care system. The term includes routine clinical or office records, records of care in any health related setting, preventive care, lifestyle evaluation, research protocols and various clinical databases. This repository of information about a single patient is generated by health care professionals as a direct result of interaction with a patient or with individuals who have personal knowledge of the patient.

- The primary patient record is the record that is used by health care professionals while providing patient care services to review patient data or document their own observations, actions, or instructions.

- The secondary patient record is a record that is derived from the primary record and contains selected data elements to aid non clinical persons in supporting, evaluating and advancing patient care. Patient care support refers to administration, regulation, and payment functions.

Practices

Methods to Ensure Data Quality

The accuracy of data depends on the manual or computer information system design for collecting, recording, storing, processing, accessing and displaying data as well as the ability and follow-through of the people involved in each phase of these activities. Everyone involved with documenting or using health information is responsible for its quality. According to AHIMA's Data Quality Management Model, there are four key processes for data:

1. Application: the purpose for which the data are collected.

2. Collection: the processes by which data elements are accumulated.

3. Warehousing: the processes and systems used to store and maintain data and data journals.

4. Analysis: the process of translating data into information utilized for an application.

Each aspect is analyzed with 10 different data characteristics:

1. Accuracy: Data are the correct values and are valid.

2. Accessibility: Data items should be easily obtainable and legal to collect.

3. Comprehensiveness: All required data items are included. Ensure that the entire scope of the data is collected and document intentional limitations.

4. Consistency: The value of the data should be reliable and the same across applications.

5. Currency: The data should be up to date. A datum value is up to date if it is current for a specific point in time. It is outdate if it was current at some preceding time yet incorrect at a later time.

6. Definition: Clear definitions should be provided so that current and future data users will know what the data mean. Each data element should have clear meaning and acceptable values.

7. Granularity: The attributes and values of data should be defined at the correct level of detail.

8. Precision: Data values should be just large enough to support the application or process.

9. Relevancy: The data are meaningful to the performance of the process or application for which they are collected.

10. Timeliness: Timeliness is determined by how the data are being used and their context.

Health Information Professionals

HIM is a very broad and successful field for health care professionals. There are several career opportunities in Health Information Management and many different traditional and non-traditional settings for an HIM professional to work within.

- Traditional settings include: Managing an HIM medical records department, cancer registry, coding, trauma registry, transcription, quality improvement, release of information, patient admissions, compliance auditor, physician accreditation, utilization review, physician offices and risk management.

- Non-traditional settings include: consulting firms, government agencies, law firms, insurance companies, correctional facilities, extended care facilities, pharmaceutical research, information technology and medical software companies.

Health Information Managers

Professional health information managers manage and construct health information programs to guarantee they accommodate medical, legal, and ethical standards. They play a crucial role in the maintenance, collection, and analyzing of data that is received by doctors, nurses, and other healthcare players. In return these healthcare data contributors rely on the information to deliver quality healthcare. Managers must work with a group of information technicians to guarantee that the patient's medical records are accurate and are available when needed.

In the United States, health information managers are typically certified as a Registered Health Information Administrator (RHIA) after achieving a bachelor's degree in health informatics or health information management from a school accredited by the Commission on Accreditation for Health Informatics and Information Management Education (CAHIIM) and after passing their respective certification exam. The Certified Health Informatics Systems Professional (CHISP) certification offered by American Society of Health Informatics Managers (ASHIM) is to credit a working level IT or clinical professional who is able to support physician adoption of Health IT. A CHISP professional needs to process knowledge of the health care environment, Health IT, IT, and soft skills including communication skills.

RHIAs usually assume a managerial position that interacts with all levels of an organization that use patient data in decision making and everyday operations. They may work in a broad range of settings that span the continuum of healthcare including office based physician practices, nursing homes, home health agencies, mental health facilities, and public health agencies.

Health information managers may specialize in registry management, data management, and data quality among other areas.

Medical Records and Health Information Technicians

Medical records (MR) and Health information technicians (HIT) are described as having the following duties according to the U.S. Bureau of Labor Statistics' Occupational Outlook Handbook:

assemble patients' health information including medical history, symptoms, examination results, diagnostic tests, treatment methods, and all other healthcare provider services. Technicians organize and manage health information data by ensuring its quality, accuracy, accessibility, and security. They regularly communicate with physicians and other healthcare professionals to clarify diagnoses or to obtain additional information.

The International Labour Organization's International Standard Classification of Occupations further notes: "Occupations included in this category require knowledge of medical terminology, legal aspects of health information, health data standards, and computer- or paper-based data management as obtained through formal education and/or prolonged on-the-job training."

MRHITs usually work in hospitals. However they also work in a variety of other healthcare settings, including office based physician practices, nursing homes, home health agencies, mental health facilities, and public health agencies. Technicians who specialize in coding are called medical coders or coding specialists.

In the United States, health information technicians are certified as a Registered Health Information Technician (RHIT) after completing an associate's degree in health information technology from a school accredited by the Commission on Accreditation for Health Informatics and Information Management Education (CAHIIM) before they may take their certification exam.

Professional Organizations

- American Health Information Management Association (AHIMA)
- American Society of Health Informatics Managers (ASHIM)
- Canadian Health Information Management Association (CHIMA)
- Commission on Accreditation of Health Informatics and Information Management Education (CAHIIM)
- Healthcare Information Management and Systems Society (HIMSS)
- Health Information Management Association of Australia Limited (HIMAA)
- Institute of Health Records and Information Management (IHRIM)

Health Information Technology

Health information technology (HIT) is information technology applied to health and health care. It supports health information management across computerized systems and the secure exchange of health information between consumers, providers, payers, and quality monitors. Based on an often-cited 2008 report on a small series of studies conducted at four sites that provide ambulatory care – three U.S. medical centers and one in the Netherlands – the use of electronic health records (EHRs) was viewed as the most promising tool for improving the overall quality, safety and efficiency of the health delivery system. According to a 2006 report by the Agency for Healthcare Research and Quality, broad and consistent utilization of HIT will:

- Improve health care quality or effectiveness:

- Increase health care productivity or efficiency;

- Prevent medical errors and increase health care accuracy and procedural correctness;

- Reduce health care costs;

- Increase administrative efficiencies and healthcare work processes;

- Decrease paperwork and unproductive or idle work time;

- Extend real-time communications of health informatics among health care professionals; and

- Expand access to affordable care.

Risk-based regulatory framework for health IT September 4, 2013 the Health IT Policy Committee (HITPC) accepted and approved recommendations from the Food and Drug Administration Safety and Innovation Act (FDASIA) working group for a risk-based regulatory framework for health information technology. The Food and Drug Administration (FDA), the Office of the National Coordinator for Health IT (ONC), and Federal Communications Commission (FCC) kicked off the FDASIA workgroup of the HITPC to provide stakeholder input into a report on a risk-based regulatory framework that promotes safety and innovation and reduces regulatory duplication, consistent with section 618 of FDASIA. This provision permitted the Secretary of Health and Human Services (HHS) to form a workgroup in order to obtain broad stakeholder input from across the health care, IT, patients and innovation spectrum. The FDA, ONC, and FCC actively participated in these discussions with stakeholders from across the health care, IT, patients and innovation spectrum.

HIMSS Good Informatics Practices-GIP is aligned with FDA risk-based regulatory framework for health information technology. GIP development began in 2004 developing risk-based IT technical guidance. Today the GIP peer-review and published modules are widely used as a tool for educating Health IT professionals.

Interoperable HIT will improve individual patient care, but it will also bring many public health benefits including:

- Early detection of infectious disease outbreaks around the country;

- Improved tracking of chronic disease management;

- Evaluation of health care based on value enabled by the collection of de-identified price and quality information that can be compared.

According to an article published in the *International Journal of Medical Informatics*, health information sharing between patients and providers helps to improve diagnosis, promotes self care, and patients also know more information about their health. The use of electronic medical records (EMRs) is still scarce now but is increasing in Canada, American and British primary care. Healthcare information in EMRs are important sources for clinical, research, and policy questions. Health information privacy (HIP) and security has been a big concern for patients and providers. Studies in Europe evaluating electronic health information poses a threat to electronic medical records and exchange of personal information. Moreover, software's traceability features allow the hospitals to collect detailed information about the preparations dispensed, creating a database of every treatment that can be used for research purposes.

Concepts and Definitions

Health information technology (HIT) is "the application of information processing involving both computer hardware and software that deals with the storage, retrieval, sharing, and use of health care information, data, and knowledge for communication and decision making". Technology is a broad concept that deals with a species' usage and knowledge of tools and crafts, and how it affects a species' ability to control and adapt to its environment. However, a strict definition is elusive; "technology" can refer to material objects of use to humanity, such as machines, hardware or utensils, but can also encompass broader themes, including systems, methods of organization, and techniques. For HIT, technology represents computers and communications attributes that can be networked to build systems for moving health information. Informatics is yet another integral aspect of HIT.

Informatics refers to the science of information, the practice of information processing, and the engineering of information systems. Informatics underlies the academic investigation and practitioner application of computing and communications technology to healthcare, health education, and biomedical research. Health informatics refers to the intersection of information science, computer science, and health care. Health informatics describes the use and sharing of information within the healthcare industry with contributions from computer science, mathematics, and psychology. It deals with the resources, devices, and methods required for optimizing the acquisition, storage, retrieval, and use of information in health and biomedicine. Health informatics tools include not only computers but also clinical guidelines, formal medical terminologies, and information and communication systems. Medical informatics, nursing informatics, public health informatics, pharmacy informatics, and translational bioinformatics are subdisciplines that inform health informatics from different disciplinary perspectives. The processes and people of concern or study are the main variables.

Implementation

The Institute of Medicine's (2001) call for the use of electronic prescribing systems in all healthcare organizations by 2010 heightened the urgency to accelerate United States hospitals' adoption of CPOE systems. In 2004, President Bush signed an Executive Order titled the President's Health Information Technology Plan, which established a ten-year plan to develop and implement electronic medical record systems across the US to improve the efficiency and safety of care. According to a study by RAND Health, the US healthcare system could save more than $81 billion annually, reduce adverse healthcare events and improve the quality of care if it were to widely adopt health information technology.

The American Recovery and Reinvestment Act, signed into law in 2009 under the Obama Administration, has provided approximately $19 billion in incentives for hospitals to shift from paper to electronic medical records. Meaningful Use, as a part of the 2009 Health Information Technology for Economic and Clinical Health (HITECH) was the incentive that included over $20 billion for the implementation of HIT alone, and provided further indication of the growing consensus regarding the potential salutary effect of HIT. The American Recovery and Reinvestment Act has set aside $2 billion which will go towards programs developed by the National Coordinator and Secretary to help healthcare providers implement HIT and provide technical assistance through various regional centers. The other $17 billion in incentives comes from Medicare and Medicaid funding for those who adopt HIT before 2015. Healthcare providers who implement electronic records can receive up to $44,000 over four years in Medicare funding and $63,750 over six years in Medicaid funding. The sooner that healthcare providers adopt the system, the more funding they receive. Those who do not adopt electronic health record systems before 2015 do not receive any federal funding.

While electronic health records have potentially many advantages in terms of providing efficient and safe care, recent reports have brought to light some challenges with implementing electronic health records. The most immediate barriers for widespread adoption of this technology have been the high initial cost of implementing the new technology and the time required for doctors to train and adapt to the new system. There have also been suspected cases of fraudulent billing, where hospitals inflate their billings to Medicare. Given that healthcare providers have not reached the deadline (2015) for adopting electronic health records, it is unclear what effects this policy will have long term.

One approach to reducing the costs and promoting wider use is to develop open standards related to EHRs. In 2014 there was widespread interest in a new HL7 draft standard, Fast Healthcare Interoperability Resources (FHIR), which is designed to be open, extensible, and easier to implement, benefiting from modern web technologies.

Types of Technology

In a 2008 study about the adoption of technology in the United States, Furukawa, and colleagues classified applications for prescribing to include electronic medical records (EMR), clinical decision support (CDS), and computerized physician order entry (CPOE). They further defined applications for dispensing to include bar-coding at medication dispensing (BarD), robot for medication dispensing (ROBOT), and automated dispensing machines (ADM). They defined applications for administration to include electronic medication administration records (eMAR) and bar-coding at medication administration (BarA or BCMA).

Electronic Health Record (EHR)

US medical groups' adoption of EHR (2005)

Although the electronic health record (EHR), previously known as the electronic medical record (EMR), is frequently cited in the literature, there is no consensus about the definition. However, there is consensus that EMRs can reduce several types of errors, including those related to prescription drugs, to preventive care, and to tests and procedures. Recurring alerts remind clinicians of intervals for preventive care and track referrals and test results. Clinical guidelines for disease management have a demonstrated benefit when accessible within the electronic record during the process of treating the patient. Advances in health informatics and widespread adoption of interoperable electronic health records promise access to a patient's records at any health care site. A 2005 report noted that medical practices in the United States are encountering barriers to adopting an EHR system, such as training, costs and complexity, but the adoption rate continues to rise. Since 2002, the National Health Service of the United Kingdom has placed emphasis on introducing computers into healthcare. As of 2005, one of the largest projects for a national EHR is by the National Health Service (NHS) in the United Kingdom. The goal of the NHS is to have 60,000,000 patients with a centralized electronic health record by 2010. The plan involves a gradual roll-out commencing May 2006, providing general practices in England access to the National Programme for IT (NPfIT), the NHS component of which is known as the "Connecting for Health Programme". However, recent surveys have shown physicians' deficiencies in understanding the patient safety features of the NPfIT-approved software. A main problem in HIT adoption is mainly seen by physicians, an important stakeholder to the process of EHR. The Thorn et al. article, elicited that emergency physicians noticed that health information exchange disrupted workflow and was less desirable to use, even though the main goal of EHR is improving coordination of care. The problem was seen that exchanges did not address the needs of end users, e.g. simplicity, user-friendly interface, and speed of systems. The same finding was seen in an earlier article with the focus on CPOE and physician resistance to its use, Bhattacherjee et al.

Clinical Point of Care Technology

Computerized Provider (Physician) Order Entry

Prescribing errors are the largest identified source of preventable errors in hospitals. A 2006 report by the Institute of Medicine estimated that a hospitalized patient is exposed to a medication error each day of his or her stay. Computerized provider order entry (CPOE), also called computerized physician order entry, can reduce total medication error rates by 80%, and adverse (serious with harm to patient) errors by 55%. A 2004 survey by found that 16% of US clinics, hospitals and medical practices are expected to be utilizing CPOE within 2 years. In addition to electronic prescribing, a standardized bar code system for dispensing drugs could prevent a quarter of drug errors. Consumer information about the risks of the drugs and improved drug packaging (clear labels, avoiding similar drug names and dosage reminders) are other error-proofing measures. Despite ample evidence of the potential to reduce medication errors, competing systems of barcoding and electronic prescribing have slowed adoption of this technology by doctors and hospitals in the United States, due to concern with interoperability and compliance with future national standards. Such concerns are not inconsequential; standards for electronic prescribing for Medicare Part D conflict with regulations in many US states. And, aside from regulatory concerns, for the small-practice physician, utilizing CPOE requires a major change in practice work flow and an additional investment of time. Many physicians are not full-time hospital staff; entering orders for their hospitalized patients means taking time away from scheduled patients.

Technological Innovations, Opportunities, and Challenges

One of the rapidly growing areas of health care innovation lies in the advanced use of data science and machine learning. The key opportunities here are:

- Health Monitoring and Diagnosis;

- Medical Treatment and Patient Care;

- Pharmaceutical Research and Development;

- Clinic Performance Optimization.

Handwritten reports or notes, manual order entry, non-standard abbreviations and poor legibility lead to substantial errors and injuries, according to the Institute of Medicine (2000) report. The follow-up IOM (2004) report, *Crossing the quality chasm: A new health system for the 21st century*, advised rapid adoption of electronic patient records, electronic medication ordering, with computer- and internet-based information systems to support clinical decisions. However, many system implementations have experienced costly failures. Furthermore, there is evidence that CPOE may actually contribute to some types of adverse events and other medical errors. For example, the period immediately following CPOE implementation resulted in significant increases in reported adverse drug events in at least one study, and evidence of other errors have been reported. Collectively, these reported adverse events describe phenomena related to the disruption of the complex adaptive system resulting from poorly implemented or inadequately planned technological innovation.

Technological Iatrogenesis

Technology may introduce new sources of error. Technologically induced errors are significant and increasingly more evident in care delivery systems. Terms to describe this new area of error production include the label technological iatrogenesis for the process and e-iatrogenic for the individual error. The sources for these errors include:

- Prescriber and staff inexperience may lead to a false sense of security; that when technology suggests a course of action, errors are avoided.

- Shortcut or default selections can override non-standard medication regimens for elderly or underweight patients, resulting in toxic doses.

- CPOE and automated drug dispensing were identified as a cause of error by 84% of over 500 health care facilities participating in a surveillance system by the United States Pharmacopoeia.

- Irrelevant or frequent warnings can interrupt work flow.

Healthcare information technology can also result in iatrogenesis if design and engineering are substandard, as illustrated in a 14-part detailed analysis done at the University of Sydney.

Revenue Cycle HIT

The HIMSS Revenue Cycle Improvement Task Force was formed to prepare for the IT changes in the U.S. (e.g. the American Recovery and Reinvestment Act of 2009 (HITECH), Affordable Care

Act, 5010 (electronic exchanges), ICD-10). An important change to the revenue cycle is the international classification of diseases (ICD) codes from 9 to 10. ICD-9 codes are set up to use three to five alphanumeric codes that represent 4,000 different types of procedures, while ICD-10 uses three to seven alphanumeric codes increasing procedural codes to 70,000. ICD-9 was outdated because there were more codes than procedures available, and to document for procedures without an ICD-9 code, unspecified codes were utilized which did not fully capture the procedures or the work involved in turn affecting reimbursement. Hence, ICD-10 was introduced to simplify the procedures with unknown codes and unify the standards closer to world standards (ICD-11). One of the main parts of Revenue Cycle HIT is charge capture, it utilizes codes to capture costs for reimbursements from different payers, such as CMS.

International Comparisons Through HIT

International health system performance comparisons are important for understanding health system complexities and finding better opportunities, which can be done through health information technology. It gives policy makers the chance to compare and contrast the systems through established indicators from health information technology, as inaccurate comparisons can lead to adverse policies.

Medical Case Management

Medical case management is a collaborative process that facilitates recommended treatment plans to assure the appropriate medical care is provided to disabled, ill or injured individuals. It is a role frequently overseen by patient advocates.

It refers to the planning and coordination of health care services appropriate to achieve the goal of medical rehabilitation. Medical case management may include, but is not limited to, care assessment, including personal interview with the injured employee, and assistance in developing, implementing and coordinating a medical care plan with health care providers, as well as the employee and his/her family and evaluation of treatment results.

Medical case management requires the evaluation of a medical condition, developing and implementing a plan of care, coordinating medical resources, communicated healthcare needs to the individual, monitors an individual's progress and promotes cost-effective care.

The term also has usage in the USA health care system, referring to the case management coordination in the managed care environment

Therapeutic Behavior Management

Therapeutic behavior management (TBM) is a technology for creating a clinical environment that brings out the best in staff while generating the highest possible compliance outcomes for patients. The techniques and practices of TBM are derived from the field of applied behavior analysis, the term describing the scientific study of behavior.

The field of applied behavior analysis was clearly defined by Baer, Wolf, and Risley (1968). Its subject matter is human behavior: why we act as we do, how we acquire habits, and how we lose them or change them, if change is needed. TBM is a branch of performance management that focuses on improving patient outcomes through improved compliance.

To understand behavior, behavior analysts use the same scientific methods that the physical sciences employ: precise definition of the behavior under study, experimentation, and consistent replication of the experimental findings. Basic research in this area has been conducted for over a century, however, applied research has been conducted only since the 1950s. Business, industrial, and government applications began in the late 1960s.

Purpose

That non-compliance represents a threat to the future of patients and providers is demonstrated by the disastrous statistics related to direct costs, over use of the system, unnecessary health service provided, and needless deaths (125,000 in the US per year). Adherence to long-term therapies: evidence for action. Counseling and education models developed over the years to improve patient understanding and compliance have failed to move the needle. These models have been time tested and on the surface are straight forward, consistent, and logical. In spite of their clear appeal to *"common sense"* they are also not terribly effective. Compliance today is about the same as it was in the middle of the 5th century and in the US it is the same as in any other first world country.

The Affordable Care Act (2010) will continue to unfold and patient behavior will have a significant impact of the bottom line of care. Providers who fall below an arbitrary quality line can expect to have Medicare revenue recouped based on outcomes of care and will begin to look for ways to mitigate their risks. Developing and implementing a well-managed TBM program targeting the 50% who are non-compliant and working with them to change their behavior may represent the best path towards reducing risk.

Origins

TBM grew out of conversations between Dr. Robert E. Wright, a registered nurse and behaviorists, Aubrey Daniels, and Dr. Darnell Lattal as they looked for more efficient approaches to patient education and behavior change. From their initial conversations came a dedicated approach for developing behavior based training programs. TBM became a carefully developed method for teaching this specialized branch of performance management to health services providers, patient advocates, and family members.

Since behavior is common to everyone, TBM shows providers and patient educators how to most effectively influence their patient's behavior regardless of their level of education or understanding of their disease. While we most often think of providers changing their patients' behavior, the fact is that patients also change their providers' behavior. More fundamentally, regardless of education or status, every time we interact with others, we change and they change. Understanding this concept is central to appreciating the power we each have to change each other for good or for less than good.

TBM is a technology of behavior change that has joined with patient education and advocacy that can change not only the behavior of patients, but support staff and providers as well. In most healthcare organizations patient education is a labor-intensive, highly somewhat punishing activity for the provider or patient educator and the patients. It is an attempt to manage patient outcomes providing a sophisticated medical education. That it generally fails is evidenced by the fact that fifty percent or more of the total patient population is non-adherent to their provider's orders.

Other Compliance Programs

Other compliance systems and philosophies fail in comparison with TBM on two issues. First, compliance depends on the ability of providers to be fair and objective and to apply the standards of care to all patients. A significant portion of patient care is based on the provider's judgment and memory of the individual patient's efforts. Providers are required to pay close attention to what the patients do say and then record the observations in the plan of care. To expect that this will is generally done in any a systematic way in today's overburdened healthcare environment is quite unrealistic. Second people are patients for a short window of time and then they are who they were for the years before they needed to use health services. Past performance is the best indicator of future performance unless there is significant behavior intervention and reinforcement of the desired behavior. Dr. Ivar Lovass famously reported in the mid 1960s that all behavior returns to baseline without reinforcement. Dr. Daniels in 2010 said, "Move the baseline." The only way to move the baseline is through positive reinforcement (e.g., TBM). "Where reinforcement goes... behavior flows." (Aubrey Daniels).

Focus on Behavior

Perhaps it is too much to expect that people who are otherwise unsophisticated about their bio-physiology and the complexities associated with the disease process will stop to consider the effects of one course of action over another. The courts have determined that informed consent means that the patient has a clear understanding of the consequences of their behavior, both good and bad, and have made an "informed" decision of what needs to be done. Clearly with a 50% failure rate. in following the doctor's orders something in the message got lost in the behavior.

Within the last few years, the emphasis on outcomes and the targeting of reimbursement based on patient outcomes has become the focus of government based reimbursement systems. Where government payers go, the private sector is not far behind. Patient compliance has been a thing of concern dating back to the origins of the practice of medicine. Hippocrates warned colleagues in his time of the dangers of patients not following their directives or not being honest with their doctors. While science has progressed in ways totally unimaginable in the first century of modern medicine, the behavior of people has not. To quote the most famous current TV doctor, Greg House, "I don't ask why patients lie, I just assume they all do." People behave based upon the consequences of their actions. This is true of patients, staff and providers.

Emily Dickinson, almost a century before B.F. Skinner began to define the science of behavior, said "Behavior is what a man does, not what he thinks, feels or believes". Behavior has existed since the beginning of time. The science is relatively simple. TBM proposes that applying the laws of behavior, similarly to performance management, to staff and patients can result in a measurable impact on the outcomes of patient care.

Clinical Pathway

Clinical pathways, also known as care pathways, critical pathways, integrated care pathways or care maps, are one of the main tools used to manage the quality in healthcare concerning the standardisation of care processes. It has been shown that their implementation reduces the variability in clinical practice and improves outcomes. Clinical pathways promote organised and efficient patient care based on evidence based practice. Clinical pathways optimise outcomes in the acute care and home care settings. Generally clinical pathways refer to medical guidelines. However a single pathway may refer to guidelines on several topics in a well specified context.

Definition of Clinical Pathway

Multidisciplinary management tool based on evidence-based practice for a specific group of patients with a predictable clinical course, in which the different tasks (interventions) by the professionals involved in the patient care are defined, optimized and sequenced either by hour (ED), day (acute care) or visit (homecare). Outcomes are tied to specific interventions.

According to an article in the *Journal of Clinical Pathways*, the concept of clinical pathways has different meanings to different stakeholders. Managed care organizations often view clinical pathways in a similar way as they view care plans, in which the care provided to a patient is definitive and deliberate. Clinical pathways can range in scope from simple medication utilization to a comprehensive treatment plan. Clinical pathways aim for greater standardization of treatment regimens and sequencing as well as improved outcomes, from both a quality of life and a clinical outcomes perspective; thus fulfilling the goal of the Triple Aim.

History

The clinical pathway concept appeared for the first time at the New England Medical Center (Boston, United States) in 1985 inspired by Karen Zander and Kathleen Bower. Clinical pathways appeared as a result of the adaptation of the documents used in industrial quality management, the Standard Operating Procedures (SOPs), whose goals are:

- Improve efficiency in the use of resources.

- Finish work in a set time.

In April, 1991, VNA *FIRST*, in consultation with the Center for Case Management, Inc., South Natick, MA, developed the Home Health Care Map Tools (now called VNA FIRST Home Care Steps Protocols.)

In 2005, the telehealth clinical pathway was introduced to standardize telehealth visits and telephone calls in homecare.

In November, 2011, Eventium,LLC, a Greater Milwaukee, Wisconsin based company, acquired the assets of VNA FIRST and Innovative Healthcare Solutions.

Characteristics

Clinical pathways (integrated care pathways) can be seen as an application of process management thinking to the improvement of patient healthcare. An aim is to re-center the focus on the patient's overall journey, rather than the contribution of each specialty or caring function independently. Instead, all are emphasised to be working together, in the same way as a cross-functional team.

More than just a guideline or a protocol, a care pathway is typically crystallised in the development and use of a single all-encompassing bedside document, that will stand as an indicator of the care a patient is likely to be provided in the course of the pathway going forward; and ultimately as a single unified legal record of the care the patient has received, and the progress of their condition, as the pathway has been undertaken.

The pathway design tries to capture the foreseeable actions which will most commonly represent best practice for most patients most of the time, and include prompts for them at the appropriate time in the pathway document to ascertain whether they have been carried out, and whether results have been as expected. In this way results are recorded, and important questions and actions are not overlooked. However, pathways are typically not prescriptive; the patient's journey is an individual one, and an important part of the purpose of the pathway documents is to capture information on "variances", where due to circumstances or clinical judgment different actions have been taken, or different results unfolded. The combined variances for a sufficiently large population of patients are then analysed to identify important or systematic features, which can be used to improve the next iteration of the pathway.

Selection Criteria

The following signals may indicate that it may be useful to commit resources to establish and implement a clinical pathway for a particular condition:

- Prevalent pathology within the care setting
- Pathology with a significant risk for patients
- Pathology with a high cost for the hospital
- Predictable clinical course
- Pathology well defined and that permits homogeneous care
- Existence of recommendations of good practices or experts opinions
- Unexplained variability of care
- Possibility of obtaining professional agreement
- Multidisciplinary implementation
- Motivation by professionals to work on a specific condition

Examples

- Liverpool Care Pathway for the Dying Patient

Health Care Quality

Health care quality is a level of value provided by any health care resource, as determined by some measurement. As with quality in other fields, it is an assessment of whether something is good enough and whether it is suitable for its purpose. The goal of health care is to provide medical resources of high quality to all who need them; that is, to ensure good quality of life, to cure illnesses when possible, to extend life expectancy, and so on. Researchers use a variety of quality measures to attempt to determine health care quality, including counts of a therapy's reduction or lessening of diseases identified by medical diagnosis, a decrease in the number of risk factors which people have following preventive care, or a survey of health indicators in a population who are accessing certain kinds of care.

Definition

Health care quality is the degree to which health care services for individuals and populations increase the likelihood of desired health outcomes. Quality of care plays an important role in describing the iron triangle of health care, which defines the intricate relationships between quality, cost, and accessibility of health care within a community. Researchers measure health care quality to identify problems caused by overuse, underuse, or misuse of health resources. In 1999, the Institute of Medicine released six domains to measure and describe quality of care in health:

1. Safe – avoiding injuries to patients from care that is intended to help them.

2. Effective – avoiding overuse and misuse of care.

3. Patient-Centered – providing care that is unique to a patient's needs.

4. Timely – reducing wait times and harmful delays for patients and providers.

5. Efficient – avoiding waste of equipment, supplies, ideas and energy.

6. Equitable – providing care that does not vary across intrinsic personal characteristics.

While essential for determining the effect of health services research interventions, measuring quality of care poses some challenges due to the limited number of outcomes that are measurable. Structural measures describe the providers' ability to provide high quality care, process measures describe the actions taken to maintain or improve community health, and outcome measures describe the impact of a health care intervention. Furthermore, due to strict regulations placed on health services research, data sources are not always complete.

Assessment of health care quality may occur on two different levels: that of the individual patient and that of populations. At the level of the individual patient, or micro-level, assessment focuses on services at the point of delivery and its subsequent effects. At the population level, or macro-level, assessments of health care quality include indicators such as life expectancy, infant mortality rates, incidence, and prevalence of certain health conditions.

Quality assessments measure these indicators against an established standard. The measures can be difficult to define in health care. Quality assurance is distinct from quality assessment and is based on the principles of total quality management (TQM). It is a method of using quality assessment measures in a system-wide manner to deliver high-quality care that is continually improving.

Methods to Assess and Improve

The Donabedain model is a common framework for assessing health care quality and identifies three domains in which health care quality can be assessed: structure, process, and outcomes. All three domains are tightly linked and build on each other. Improvements in structure and process are often observed in outcomes. Some examples of improvements in process are: clinical practice guidelines, analysis of cost efficiency, and risk management, which consists of proactive steps to prevent medical errors.

Cost Efficiency Cost Efficiency, or cost effectiveness, determines whether the benefits of a service exceed the cost incurred to provide the service. A health care service is sometimes not cost efficient due to either overutilization or underutilization. Overutilization, or overuse, occurs when the value of health care is diluted with wasted resources. Consequently, depriving someone else of the potential benefits from obtaining the service. Costs or risks of treatment outweigh the benefits in overused health care. In contrast, underutilization, or underuse, occurs when the benefits of a treatment outweigh the risks or costs, but it is not used. There are potential adverse health outcomes with underutilization. One example is the lack of early cancer detection and treatment which leads to decreased cancer survival rates.

Critical Pathways Critical Pathways are outcome-based and patient-centered case management tools that take on an interdisciplinary approach by "facilitating coordination of care among multiple clinical departments and caregivers". Health care managers utilize critical pathways as a method to reduce variation in care, decrease resource utilization, and improve quality of care. Using critical pathways to reduce costs and errors improves quality by providing a systematic approach to assessing health care outcomes. Reducing variations in practice patterns promotes improved collaboration among interdisciplinary players in the health care system.

Health Professional Perspective

The quality of the health care given by a health professional can be judged by its outcome, the technical performance of the care and by interpersonal relationships.

"Outcome" is a change in patients' health, such as reduction in pain, relapses, or death rates. Large differences in outcomes can be measured for individual medical providers, and smaller differences can be measured by studying large groups, such as low- and high-volume doctors. Significant initiatives to improve healthcare quality outcomes have been undertaken that include clinical practice guidelines, cost efficiency, critical pathways, and risk management.

Clinical Practice Guideline "Technical performance" is the extent to which a health professional conformed to the best practices established by medical guidelines. Clinical practice guidelines, or medical practice guidelines, are scientifically based protocols to assist providers in adopting a "best practice" approach in delivering care for a given health condition. Standardizing the practice of medicine improves quality of care by concurrently promoting lower costs and better outcomes. The presumption is providers following medical guidelines are giving the best care and give the most hope of a good outcome. Technical performance is judged from a quality perspective without regard to the actual outcome - so for example, if a physician gives care according to the guidelines but a patient's health does not improve, then by this measure, the quality of the "technical performance" is still high.

Risk Management Risk management consists of "proactive efforts to prevent adverse events related to clinical care" and is focused on avoiding medical malpractice. Health care professionals are not immune to lawsuits; therefore, health care organizations have taken initiatives to establish protocols specifically to reduce malpractice litigation. Malpractice concerns can result in defensive medicine, or threat of malpractice litigation, which can compromise patient safety and care by inducing additional testing or treatments. One widely used form of defensive medicine is ordering costly imaging which can be wasteful. However, other defensive behaviors may actually reduce access to care and pose risks of physical harm. Many specialty physicians report doing more for patients, such as using unnecessary diagnostic tests, because of malpractice risks. In turn, it is especially crucial that risk management approaches employ principles of cost efficiency with standardized practice guidelines and critical pathways.

Patient Perspective

Patient satisfaction surveys are the main qualitative measure of the patient perspective. Patients may not have the clinical judgement of physicians and often judge quality on the basis of practitioner's concern and demeanor, among other things. As a result, patient satisfaction surveys have become a somewhat controversial measure of quality care. Proponents argue that patient surveys can provide needed feedback to physicians to assist on improving their practice. In addition, patient satisfaction often correlates with patient involvement in decision making and can improve patient-centered care. Patients' evaluation of care can identify opportunities for improvement in care, reducing costs, monitoring performance of health plans, and provide a comparison across health care institutions. Opponents of patient satisfaction surveys are often unconvinced that the data is reliable, that the expense does not justify the costs, and that what is measured is not a good indicator of quality.

The Department of Health and Human Services bases 30 percent of hospitals' Medicare reimbursement on patient satisfaction survey scores on a survey, known as the Hospital Consumer Assessment of Healthcare Providers and Systems (HCAHPS). "Beginning in October 2012, the Affordable Care Act implemented a policy that withholds 1 percent of total Medicare reimbursements—approximately $850 million—from hospitals (that percentage will double in 2017). Each year, only hospitals with high patient-satisfaction scores and a measure of certain basic care standards will earn that money back, and top performers receive bonuses from the pool."

History in the United States

As early as the 19th century, healthcare quality improvement interventions were implemented in an effort to improve healthcare outcomes. Healthcare quality improvement further developed in the 1900s, with notable improvements for the modern field of quality improvement taking place in the late 1960s.

In the early 1900s, Dr. Ernest Codman of Massachusetts General Hospital suggested a measure that tracked each patient of the hospital to determine effectiveness of their treatment. His proposal of a system to track patient care to determine quality and standard of hospital care dubbed him one of the earliest advocates of healthcare quality. Shortly after, influenced by the work of Dr. Codman, the American College of Surgeons (ACS) was founded. In 1918, the ACS developed the Minimum Standard for Hospitals, which was one page. As a result of the 1918 Minimum Standard for Hospitals, ACS began performing on-site inspections of hospitals to determine if they were up to par. During the first on-site inspections of 692 hospitals, only 13% met the minimum standard.

In 1945, Joseph Juran and Edwards Deming established Quality Improvement (QI) as a formal approach to analyzing systematic efforts to improve performance. Specifically, Deming, a philosopher, placed emphasis on the macro level of organizational management and improvement via a systems approach. Juran, on the other hand, strategized quality planning, control, and improvement at the micro level. He encouraged questions, believing they deepened understanding of problems and led to increased effectiveness in planning and taking action. Together, their work influenced quality of both American public and private organizations in fields from healthcare and industry to government and education.

The Joint Commission on Accreditation of Hospitals (JCAH) was established in 1951 as an independent and non-profit organization that provided voluntary accreditation to hospitals that met minimum quality standards. JCAH was formed by the combined forces of the American College of Physicians, the American College of Surgeons, the American Hospital Association, the American Medical Association, and the Canadian Medical Association. In 1952, the ACS formally transferred its Hospital Standardization Program to JCAH. JCAH began to charge a fee for surveys in 1964.

The Social Security Amendments of 1965 were passed by Congress in an attempt to grant hospitals accredited by JCAH "deemed status". As such, those same hospitals were said to meet the necessary requirements to participate in Medicare and Medicaid. Until 1966, when Avedis Donabedian, MD published his "Evaluating the Quality of Medical Care", the study of health care quality was based on structure (e.g., licensing, staffing levels, accreditation). Donabedian demonstrated a new perspective on analyzing healthcare quality that was based on structure, process, and outcome.

The National Academy of Sciences established the Institute of Medicine (IOM) in 1970. The IOM, a non-profit and independent scientific advisor, was created to improve health on a national scale. The Accreditation Association for Ambulatory Health Care (AAAHC) formed in 1970 to improve healthcare quality for patients served by ambulatory health care organizations by setting standards for ambulatory healthcare accreditation, similar to JCAH. The Agency for Healthcare Research and Quality (AHRQ) was created in 1989 in order to improve quality, safety, efficiency, and effectiveness of health care through research.

In 1990, the National Committee for Quality Assurance (NCQA) was entrusted to offer accreditation programs for managed care organizations. The NCQA was established as an independent non-profit dedicated to improving health care quality through accreditation and performance measurement. In 1991, Dr. Don Berwick's non-profit Institute for Healthcare Improvement (IHI) was founded. Rather than only focus on national health care quality improvement, IHI campaigned but nationally and worldwide. Directing the focus onto the patient as a consumer, the National Patient Safety Foundation was established in 1996. In 1998, by presidential directive, the Quality Interagency Coordination Task Force (QuIC) was created to increase coordination of federal agencies that work toward improving quality care. When the IOM published *To Err is Human* in 1999, revealing high medical error mortality rates, the QuIC published a report that inventoried regulatory and legislative initiatives that sought to improve issues surrounding medical error. Also in 1999, the National Quality Forum was founded. The private, non-profit forum aims to standardize health care delivery and measurements of quality. In response to the patient safety concerns discussed in *To Err is Human*, the United States enacted the Patient Safety and Quality Improvement Act in 2005.

More recently, the focus of quality improvement has been emerging health information technology (e.g., electronic health records and patient-centered care. As a result, the formation of Patient-Centered Medical Homes (PCMH) began to gain popularity in 2007. Under PCMH, care among personal primary care physicians and specialists increased coordination and integration of care for the patient. Furthermore, technology was used to maintain personal health information and enhance quality and safety. Since 2007, various studies have demonstrated the wide array of benefits of PCMHs in healthcare quality improvement.

Organizations which Determine Quality

Organizations which work to set standards and measures for health care quality include Government health systems; private health systems, accreditation programs such as those for hospital accreditation, health associations, or those who wish to establish international healthcare accreditation; philanthropic foundations; and health research institutions. These organizations seek to define the concept of quality in healthcare, measure that quality, and then encourage the regular measurement of quality so as to provide evidence that health interventions are effective.

In the United States

Multiple organizations have established measures to define quality since providers, patients and payers have different views and expectations of quality. This complex situation creates a challenge because most often the measures of quality are not comparable across organizations and there are issues of transferability and merging across systems. Consequently, while measuring health care quality for these reasons, high quality longitudinal provides a substantive framework from which health services researchers can work.

The Centers for Medicare and Medicaid Services (CMS) designs quality evaluations, collects quality, and manages funding for the central government Medicare and Medicaid programs. In 2001, CMS started multiple quality initiatives including, but not limited to: the Home Health Quality Initiative, the Hospital Value-based Purchasing Program, the Hospice Quality Reporting Program, the Inpatient Rehabilitation Facilities Quality Reporting, and the Long-Term Care Hospitals Quality Reporting. CMS established initiatives to measure and improve the quality of care for Medicaid and CHIP beneficiaries for services provided under the umbrella of Early Periodic Screening, Diagnosis, and Treatment Program (EPSDT), including maternal and infant health, home and community-based services, preventative care, health disparities, patient safety, external quality review, and improving care transitions. For broader quality control, CMS also created Hospital Compare, which is a large public reporting program that measures and also reports processes of care and outcomes for various health care interventions including heart failure, pneumonia, and acute myocardial infarction.

The Agency for Healthcare Research and Quality (AHRQ) is a central government organization which collects public reports of health quality evaluation to increase the safety and quality of health care. AHRQ works together with the United States Department of Health and Human Services to make ensure that evidence is understood and used by the medical communities to elevate the quality of care. To fulfill its mission, AHRQ contracts with several subsites.

CMS and AHRQ have collectively established the Hospital Consumer Assessment of Healthcare Providers and Systems (CAHPS) survey. The CAHPS survey collects uniform measures of patients' perspectives on various aspects of the care they receive in inpatient settings. The results are published on the Hospital Compare website, which may be used by health care organizations and researchers to improve the quality of their services. Purchasers, consumers, and researchers may also use the data to make informed business choices.

The Joint Commission Accreditation for Healthcare Organization (JCAHO) is a nonprofit organization that assesses quality at multiple levels by inspecting health care facilities for adherence to clinical guidelines, compliance with rules and regulations for medical staff skills and qualifications, review of medical records to evaluate care processes and search for medical errors, and inspects buildings for safety code violations. JCAHO also provides feedback and opportunities for improvement, while simultaneously issuing citations for closures of facilities deemed noncompliant with set measures of quality standards.

In the United Kingdom

In the UK, healthcare is publicly funded and delivered through the National Health Service (NHS) and quality is overseen by a number of different bodies. Monitor, a non-departmental public body sponsored by the Department of Health, is the sector regulator for health services in England. It works closely with the Care Quality Commission (CQC) a government-funded independent body responsible for overseeing the quality and safety of health and social care services in England, including hospitals, care homes, dental and GPs and other care services.

Medical professions in the UK also have their own membership and regulatory associations. These include the General Medical Council (GMC), the Nursing and Midwifery Council, the General Dental Council and the Health and Care Professions Council. Other healthcare quality organisations include the Healthcare Quality Improvement Partnership (HQIP), a charity and limited company established by the Academy of Medical Royal Colleges, the Royal College of Nursing, National Voices; and Healthwatch, a statutory national body that works with groups across the country to ensure that patients' views are at the heart of decisions about the healthcare system.

A number of health think tanks, including the King's Fund, the Nuffield Trust and the Health Foundation also offer analysis, resources and commentary around healthcare quality. In 2013, the Nuffield Trust and the Health Foundation launched QualityWatch, an independent research programme tracking how healthcare quality in England is changing in response to rising remand and limited funding.

In India

International India healthcare quality is managed by NABH National Accreditation Board for Healthcare providers.Renowned healthcare quality experts are Dr.Mahboob ali khan who has published many publications related to improving healthcare quality management in India.

References

- Panella, M (2003). "Reducing clinical variations with clinical pathways: do pathways work?". Int J Qual Health Care. 15 (6): 509–521. doi:10.1093/intqhc/mzg057. Retrieved 27 July 2014

- Boaden, Ruth; Nathan Proudlove; Melanie Wilson (1999). "An exploratory study of bed management". Journal of Management in Medicine. 13 (4): 234–50. doi:10.1108/02689239910292945. ISSN 0268-9235. PMID 10787495

- Peter R. Kongstvedt, "The Managed Health Care Handbook," Fourth Edition, Aspen Publishers, Inc., 2001, page 788 ISBN 0-8342-1726-0

- "Patient Experience". Bed management: Review of National Findings. Audit Commission. 2003-06-19. Retrieved 2008-05-20

- Jha, A. K., Doolan, D., Grandt, D., Scott, T. & Bates, D. W. (2008). The use of health information technology in seven nations. International Journal of Medical Informatics, corrected proof in-press

- "The NHS: Has the Additional Funding Worked?". Civitas. April 2005. pp. 2–3. Archived from the original on 2008-08-28. Retrieved 2008-05-20

- Campbell, E. M., Sittig, D. F., Ash, J. S., Guappone, K. P., & Dykstra, R. H. (2007). In reply to: "e-Iatrogenesis: The most critical consequence of CPOE and other HIT. Journal of the American Medical Informatics Association

- Mayhew, Les; Smith, David (December 2006). Latest research statistically proves A&E waiting times are not being met (PDF). Using queuing theory to analyse completion times in accident and emergency departments in the light of the Government 4-hour target. Cass Business School. ISBN 978-1-905752-06-5. Retrieved 2008-05-20

- Healthcare Integration and Connectivity: Results of a Survey by the Enterprise Information Systems Steering Committee page 4. HIMSS. Retrieved 1/8/2010

- Bradley, V. M., Steltenkamp, C. L., & Hite, K. B. (2006). Evaluation of reported medication errors before and after implementation of computerized practitioner order entry. Journal Healthc Inf Manag, 20(4): 46-53

- Santell, John P (2004). "Computer Related Errors: What Every Pharmacist Should Know" (PDF). United States Pharmacopia. Retrieved 2006-06-20

- Baer, D.M., Wolf, M.M., & Risley, T.R., (1968). Some current dimensions of applied behavior analysis. Journal of Applied Behavior Analysis, 1, 91-97

4

Health Care System: An Integrated Study

A group of people or institutions that focus on meeting the demands of health care are a part of the health system. Universal health care is a health care system in which a country's citizens are promised medical aid as well as financial guarantee. The aspects elucidated in this chapter are of vital importance, and provide a better understanding of health care.

Health System

A health system, also sometimes referred to as health care system or as healthcare system, is the organization of people, institutions, and resources that deliver health care services to meet the health needs of target populations.

There is a wide variety of health systems around the world, with as many histories and organizational structures as there are nations. Implicitly, nations must design and develop health systems in accordance with their needs and resources, although common elements in virtually all health systems are primary healthcare and public health measures. In some countries, health system planning is distributed among market participants. In others, there is a concerted effort among governments, trade unions, charities, religious organizations, or other co-ordinated bodies to deliver planned health care services targeted to the populations they serve. However, health care planning has been described as often evolutionary rather than revolutionary.

Goals

The World Health Organization (WHO), the directing and coordinating authority for health within the United Nations system, is promoting a goal of universal health care: to ensure that all people obtain the health services they need without suffering financial hardship when paying for them. According to WHO, healthcare systems' goals are good health for the citizens, responsiveness to the expectations of the population, and fair means of funding operations. Progress towards them depends on how systems carry out four vital functions: provision of health care services, resource generation, financing, and stewardship. Other dimensions for the evaluation of health systems include quality, efficiency, acceptability, and equity. They have also been described in the United States as "the five C's": Cost, Coverage, Consistency, Complexity, and Chronic Illness. Also, continuity of health care is a major goal.

Definitions

Often health system has been defined with a reductionist perspective, for example reducing it to healthcare system. In many publications, for example, both expressions are used interchangeably.

Some authors have developed arguments to expand the concept of health systems, indicating additional dimensions that should be considered:

- Health systems should not be expressed in terms of their components only, but also of their interrelationships;

- Health systems should include not only the institutional or supply side of the health system, but also the population;

- Health systems must be seen in terms of their goals, which include not only health improvement, but also equity, responsiveness to legitimate expectations, respect of dignity, and fair financing, among others;

- Health systems must also be defined in terms of their functions, including the direct provision of services, whether they are medical or public health services, but also "other enabling functions, such as stewardship, financing, and resource generation, including what is probably the most complex of all challenges, the health workforce."

World Health Organization Definition

The World Health Organization defines health systems as follows:

A health system consists of all organizations, people and actions whose primary intent is to promote, restore or maintain health. This includes efforts to influence determinants of health as well as more direct health-improving activities. A health system is therefore more than the pyramid of publicly owned facilities that deliver personal health services. It includes, for example, a mother caring for a sick child at home; private providers; behaviour change programmes; vector-control campaigns; health insurance organizations; occupational health and safety legislation. It includes inter-sectoral action by health staff, for example, encouraging the ministry of education to promote female education, a well known determinant of better health.

Providers

Healthcare providers are institutions or individuals providing healthcare services. Individuals including health professionals and allied health professions can be self-employed or working as an employee in a hospital, clinic, or other health care institution, whether government operated, private for-profit, or private not-for-profit (e.g. non-governmental organization). They may also work outside of direct patient care such as in a government health department or other agency, medical laboratory, or health training institution. Examples of health workers are doctors, nurses, midwives, dietitians, paramedics, dentists, medical laboratory technologists, therapists, psychologists, pharmacists, chiropractors, optometrists, community health workers, traditional medicine practitioners, and others.

Financial Resources

There are generally five primary methods of funding health systems:

1. general taxation to the state, county or municipality

2. national health insurance

3. voluntary or private health insurance

4. out-of-pocket payments

5. donations to charities

Most countries' systems feature a mix of all five models. One study based on data from the OECD concluded that all types of health care finance "are compatible with" an efficient health system. The study also found no relationship between financing and cost control.

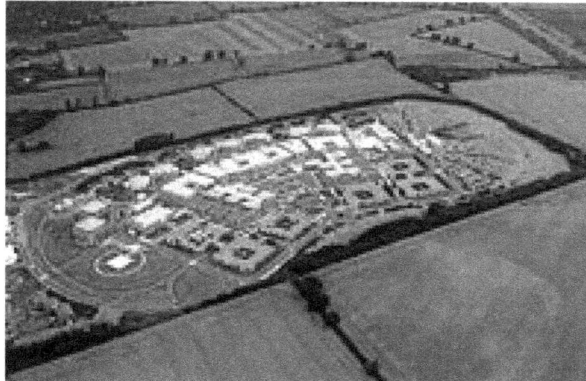

Norfolk and Norwich University Hospital, a National Health Service hospital in the United Kingdom.

The term health insurance is generally used to describe a form of insurance that pays for medical expenses. It is sometimes used more broadly to include insurance covering disability or long-term nursing or custodial care needs. It may be provided through a social insurance program, or from private insurance companies. It may be obtained on a group basis (e.g., by a firm to cover its employees) or purchased by individual consumers. In each case premiums or taxes protect the insured from high or unexpected health care expenses.

By estimating the overall cost of health care expenses, a routine finance structure (such as a monthly premium or annual tax) can be developed, ensuring that money is available to pay for the health care benefits specified in the insurance agreement. The benefit is typically administered by a government agency, a non-profit health fund or a corporation operating seeking to make a profit.

Many forms of commercial health insurance control their costs by restricting the benefits that are paid by through deductibles, co-payments, coinsurance, policy exclusions, and total coverage limits and will severely restrict or refuse coverage of pre-existing conditions. Many government schemes also have co-payment schemes but exclusions are rare because of political pressure. The larger insurance schemes may also negotiate fees with providers.

Many forms of social insurance schemes control their costs by using the bargaining power of their community they represent to control costs in the health care delivery system. For example, by negotiating drug prices directly with pharmaceutical companies negotiating standard fees with the medical profession, or reducing unnecessary health care costs. Social schemes sometimes feature contributions related to earnings as part of a scheme to deliver universal health care, which may or may not also involve the use of commercial and non-commercial insurers. Essentially the more wealthy pay proportionately more into the scheme to cover the needs of the relatively poor who therefore contribute proportionately less. There are usually caps on the contributions of the wealthy and minimum payments that must be made by the insured (often in the form of a minimum contribution, similar to a deductible in commercial insurance models).

In addition to these traditional health care financing methods, some lower income countries and development partners are also implementing non-traditional or innovative financing mechanisms for scaling up delivery and sustainability of health care, such as micro-contributions, public-private partnerships, and market-based financial transaction taxes. For example, as of June 2011, UNITAID had collected more than one billion dollars from 29 member countries, including several from Africa, through an air ticket solidarity levy to expand access to care and treatment for HIV/AIDS, tuberculosis and malaria in 94 countries.

Payment Models

In most countries, wage costs for healthcare practitioners are estimated to represent between 65% and 80% of renewable health system expenditures. There are three ways to pay medical practitioners: fee for service, capitation, and salary. There has been growing interest in blending elements of these systems.

Fee-for-service

Fee-for-service arrangements pay general practitioners (GPs) based on the service. They are even more widely used for specialists working in ambulatory care.

There are two ways to set fee levels:

- By individual practitioners.

- Central negotiations (as in Japan, Germany, Canada and in France) or hybrid model (such as in Australia, France's sector 2, and New Zealand) where GPs can charge extra fees on top of standardized patient reimbursement rates.

Capitation

In *capitation payment systems*, GPs are paid for each patient on their "list", usually with adjustments for factors such as age and gender. According to OECD, "these systems are used in Italy (with some fees), in all four countries of the United Kingdom (with some fees and allowances for specific services), Austria (with fees for specific services), Denmark (one third of income with remainder fee for service), Ireland (since 1989), the Netherlands (fee-for-service for privately insured patients and public employees) and Sweden (from 1994). Capitation payments have become more frequent in "managed care" environments in the United States."

According to OECD, "Capitation systems allow funders to control the overall level of primary health expenditures, and the allocation of funding among GPs is determined by patient registrations. However, under this approach, GPs may register too many patients and under-serve them, select the better risks and refer on patients who could have been treated by the GP directly. Freedom of consumer choice over doctors, coupled with the principle of "money following the patient" may moderate some of these risks. Aside from selection, these problems are likely to be less marked than under salary-type arrangements."

Salary Arrangements

In several OECD countries, general practitioners (GPs) are employed on *salaries* for the government. According to OECD, "Salary arrangements allow funders to control primary care costs directly; however, they may lead to under-provision of services (to ease workloads), excessive referrals to secondary providers and lack of attention to the preferences of patients." There has been movement away from this system.

Information Resources

Sound information plays an increasingly critical role in the delivery of modern health care and efficiency of health systems. Health informatics – the intersection of information science, medicine and healthcare – deals with the resources, devices, and methods required to optimize the acquisition and use of information in health and biomedicine. Necessary tools for proper health information coding and management include clinical guidelines, formal medical terminologies, and computers and other information and communication technologies. The kinds of data processed may include patients' medical records, hospital administration and clinical functions, and human resources information.

The use of health information lies at the root of evidence-based policy and evidence-based management in health care. Increasingly, information and communication technologies are being utilised to improve health systems in developing countries through: the standardisation of health information; computer-aided diagnosis and treatment monitoring; informing population groups on health and treatment.

Management

The management of any health system is typically directed through a set of policies and plans adopted by government, private sector business and other groups in areas such as personal healthcare delivery and financing, pharmaceuticals, health human resources, and public health.

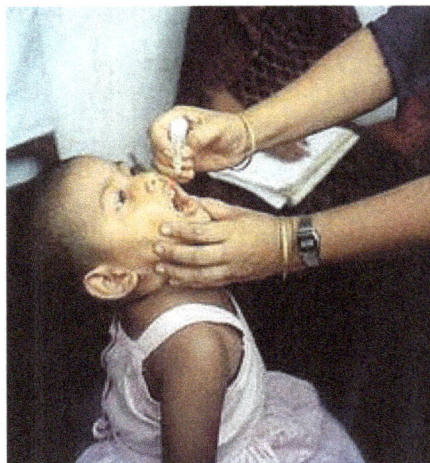

A child being immunized against polio.

Public health is concerned with threats to the overall health of a community based on population health analysis. The population in question can be as small as a handful of people, or as large as all the inhabitants of several continents (for instance, in the case of a pandemic). Public health is typically divided into epidemiology, biostatistics and health services. Environmental, social, behavioral, and occupational health are also important subfields.

Today, most governments recognize the importance of public health programs in reducing the incidence of disease, disability, the effects of ageing and health inequities, although public health generally receives significantly less government funding compared with medicine. For example, most countries have a vaccination policy, supporting public health programs in providing vaccinations to promote health. Vaccinations are voluntary in some countries and mandatory in some countries. Some governments pay all or part of the costs for vaccines in a national vaccination schedule.

The rapid emergence of many chronic diseases, which require costly long-term care and treatment, is making many health managers and policy makers re-examine their healthcare delivery practices. An important health issue facing the world currently is HIV/AIDS. Another major public health concern is diabetes. In 2006, according to the World Health Organization, at least 171 million people worldwide suffered from diabetes. Its incidence is increasing rapidly, and it is estimated that by the year 2030, this number will double. A controversial aspect of public health is the control of tobacco smoking, linked to cancer and other chronic illnesses.

Antibiotic resistance is another major concern, leading to the reemergence of diseases such as tuberculosis. The World Health Organization, for its World Health Day 2011 campaign, is calling for intensified global commitment to safeguard antibiotics and other antimicrobial medicines for future generations.

Health Systems Performance

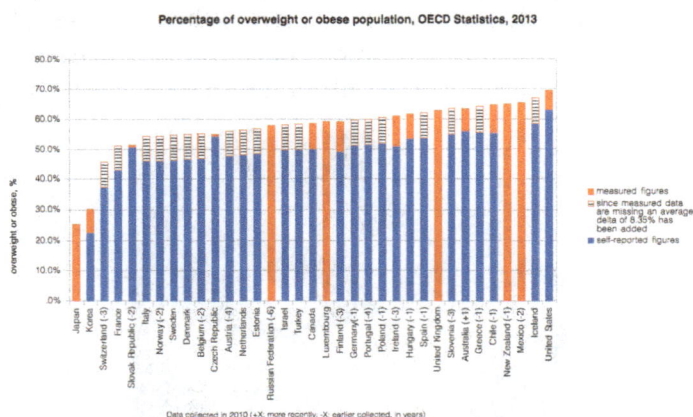

Percentage of overweight or obese population in 2010

Since 2000, more and more initiatives have been taken at the international and national levels in order to strengthen national health systems as the core components of the global health system. Having this scope in mind, it is essential to have a clear, and unrestricted, vision of national health systems that might generate further progresses in global health. The elaboration and the selection of performance indicators are indeed both highly dependent on the conceptual framework adopted for the evaluation of the health systems performances. Like most social systems, health systems are complex adaptive systems where change does not necessarily follow rigid epidemiological models. In complex systems path dependency, emergent properties and other non-linear patterns are under-explored and unmeasured, which can lead to the development of inappropriate guidelines for developing responsive health systems.

An increasing number of tools and guidelines are being published by international agencies and development partners to assist health system decision-makers to monitor and assess health systems strengthening including human resources development using standard definitions, indicators and measures. In response to a series of papers published in 2012 by members of the World Health Organization's Task Force on Developing Health Systems Guidance, researchers from the Future Health Systems consortium argue that there is insufficient focus on the 'policy implementation gap'. Recognizing the diversity of stakeholders and complexity of health systems is crucial to ensure that evidence-based guidelines are tested with requisite humility and without a rigid adherence to models dominated by a limited number of disciplines.

Health Policy and Systems Research (HPSR) is an emerging multidisciplinary field that challenges 'disciplinary capture' by dominant health research traditions, arguing that these traditions generate premature and inappropriately narrow definitions that impede rather than enhance health systems strengthening. HPSR focuses on low- and middle-income countries and draws on the relativist social science paradigm which recognises that all phenomena are constructed through human behaviour and interpretation. In using this approach, HPSR offers insight into health systems by generating a complex understanding of context in order to enhance health policy learning. HPSR calls for greater involvement of local actors, including policy makers, civil society and researchers, in decisions that are made around funding health policy research and health systems strengthening.

International Comparisons

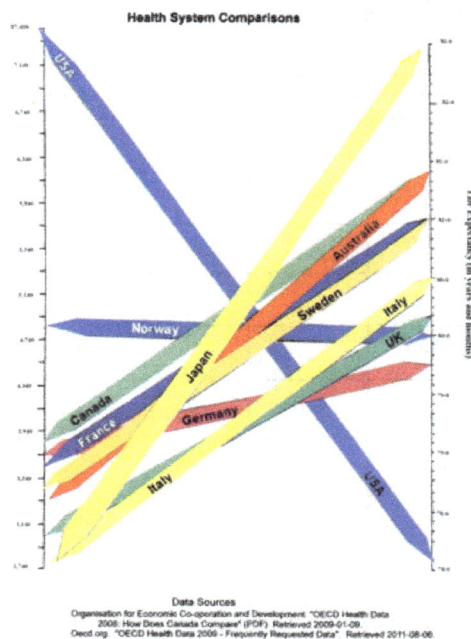

Chart comparing 2008 health care spending (left) vs. life expectancy (right) in OECD countries.

Health systems can vary substantially from country to country, and in the last few years, comparisons have been made on an international basis. The World Health Organization, in its *World Health Report 2000*, provided a ranking of health systems around the world according to criteria of the overall level and distribution of health in the populations, and the responsiveness and fair financing of health care services. The goals for health systems, according to the WHO's *World Health Report 2000 – Health systems: improving performance* (WHO, 2000), are good health, responsiveness to the expectations of the population, and fair financial contribution. There have been several debates around the results of this WHO exercise, and especially based on the country ranking linked to it, insofar as it appeared to depend mostly on the choice of the retained indicators.

Direct comparisons of health statistics across nations are complex. The Commonwealth Fund, in its annual survey, "Mirror, Mirror on the Wall", compares the performance of the health systems in Australia, New Zealand, the United Kingdom, Germany, Canada and the United States Its 2007 study found that, although the United States system is the most expensive, it consistently underperforms compared to the other countries. A major difference between the United States and the other countries in the study is that the United States is the only country without universal health care. The OECD also collects comparative statistics, and has published brief country profiles. Health Consumer Powerhouse makes comparisons between both national health care systems in the Euro health consumer index and specific areas of health care such as diabetes or hepatitis.

Country	Life expectancy	Infant mortality rate	Preventable deaths per 100,000 people in 2007	Physicians per 1000 people	Nurses per 1000 people	Per capita expenditure on health (USD PPP)	Health-care costs as a percent of GDP	% of government revenue spent on health	% of health costs paid by government
Australia	81.4	4.49	57	2.8	10.1	3,353	8.5	17.7	67.5
Canada	81.4	4.78	77	2.2	9.0	3,844	10.0	16.7	70.2
France	81.0	3.34	55	3.3	7.7	3,679	11.0	14.2	78.3
Germany	79.8	3.48	76	3.5	10.5	3,724	10.4	17.6	76.4
Italy	82.1	3.33	60	4.2	6.1	2,771	8.7	14.1	76.6
Japan	82.6	2.17	61	2.1	9.4	2,750	8.2	16.8	80.4
Norway	80.0	3.47	64	3.8	16.2	4,885	8.9	17.9	84.1
Sweden	81.0	2.73	61	3.6	10.8	3,432	8.9	13.6	81.4
United Kingdom	80.1	4.5	83	2.5	9.5	3,051	8.4	15.8	81.3
United States	78.1	5.9	96	2.4	10.6	7,437	16.0	18.5	45.1

Physicians and hospital beds per 1000 inhabitants vs Health Care Spending in 2008 for OECD Countries.

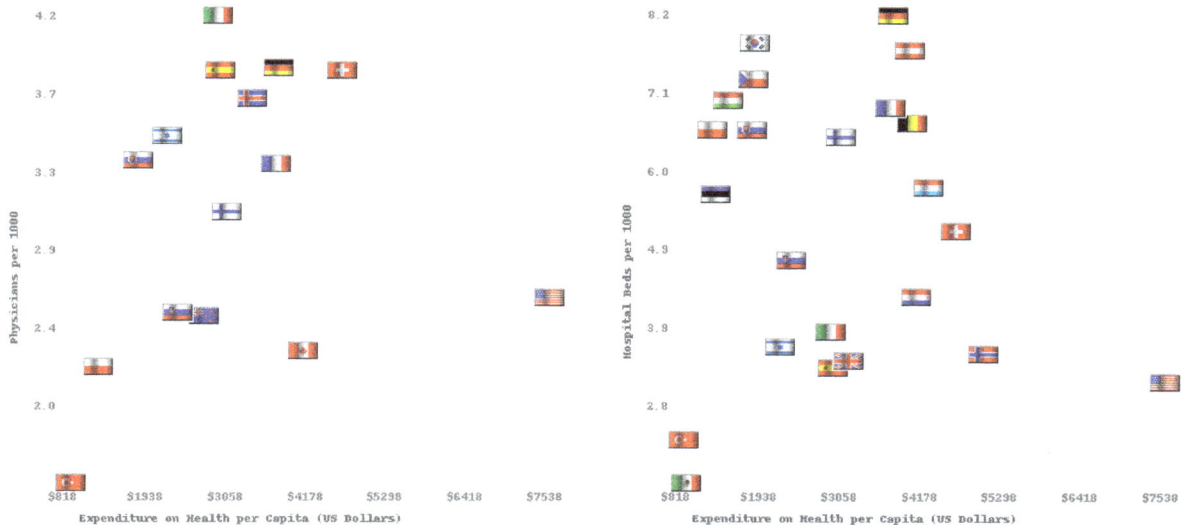

Physicians per 1000 / Expenditure on Health per Capita (US Dollars)

Hospital Beds per 1000 / Expenditure on Health per Capita (US Dollars)

Single-payer Healthcare

Single-payer healthcare is a healthcare system in which the state, financed by taxes, covers basic healthcare costs for all residents regardless of income, occupation, or health status. The alternatives include "multi-payer" systems in which private individuals or their employers buy health insurance or healthcare services from private or public providers.

Single-payer systems may contract for healthcare services from private organizations (as is the case in Canada) or may own and employ healthcare resources and personnel (as is the case in the United Kingdom). "Single-payer" describes the mechanism by which healthcare is paid for by a single public authority, not the type of delivery or for whom physicians work. In contrast, multi-payer healthcare uses a mixed public-private system.

Description

Single-payer health healthcare collects all medical fees and then pays for all services, by a single government (or government-related) source. In wealthy nations, that kind of publicly managed insurance is typically extended to all citizens and legal residents. Examples include the United Kingdom's National Health Service, Australia's Medicare, Canada's Medicare, and Taiwan's National Health Insurance.

The standard usage of the term "single-payer healthcare" refers to health insurance, as opposed to healthcare delivery, operating as a public service and offered to citizens and legal residents towards providing nearly universal or universal healthcare. The fund can be managed by the government directly or as a publicly owned and regulated agency. Some writers describe publicly administered systems as "single-payer plans". Some writers have described any system of healthcare which intends to cover the entire population, such as voucher plans, as "single-payer plans".

Countries with Single-payer Systems

Various nations worldwide have single-payer health insurance programs. These programs generally provide some form of universal healthcare, which are implemented in a variety of ways. In some cases doctors are employed, and hospitals run by, the government such as in the United Kingdom or Spain. Alternatively the government may purchase healthcare services from outside organizations, such as the approach taken in Canada.

Canada

Healthcare in Canada is delivered through a publicly funded healthcare system, which is mostly free at the point of use and has most services provided by private entities. The system was established by the provisions of the Canada Health Act of 1984. The government assures the quality of care through federal standards. The government does not participate in day-to-day care or collect any information about an individual's health, which remains confidential between a person and his or her physician. Canada's provincially based Medicare systems are cost-effective partly because of their administrative simplicity. In each province, each doctor handles the insurance claim against the provincial insurer. There is no need for the person who accesses healthcare to be involved in billing and reclaim. Private insurance represents a minimal part of the overall system.

Competitive practices such as advertising are kept to a minimum, thus maximizing the percentage of revenues that go directly towards care. In general, costs are paid through funding from income taxes, except in British Columbia, the only province to impose a fixed monthly premium which is waived or reduced for those on low incomes. There are no deductibles on basic health care and co-pays are extremely low or non-existent (supplemental insurance such as Fair Pharmacare may have deductibles, depending on income). A health card is issued by the Provincial Ministry of Health to each individual who enrolls for the program and everyone receives the same level of care. There is no need for a variety of plans because virtually all essential basic care is covered, including maternity and infertility problems. Depending on the province, dental and vision care may not be covered but are often insured by employers through private companies. In some provinces, private supplemental plans are available for those who desire private rooms if they are hospitalized. Cosmetic surgery and some forms of elective surgery are not considered essential care and are generally not covered. These can be paid out-of-pocket or through private insurers. Health coverage is not affected by loss or change of jobs, as long as premiums are up to date, and there are no lifetime limits or exclusions for pre-existing conditions.

Pharmaceutical medications are covered by public funds for the elderly or indigent, or through employment-based private insurance. Drug prices are negotiated with suppliers by the federal government to control costs. Family physicians (often known as general practitioners or GPs in Canada) are chosen by individuals. If a patient wishes to see a specialist or is counseled to see a specialist, a referral can be made by a GP. Canadians do wait for some treatments and diagnostic services. Survey data shows that the median wait time to see a special physician is a little over four weeks with 89.5% waiting less than three months. The median wait time for diagnostic services such as MRI and CAT scans is two weeks, with 86.4% waiting less than three months. The median wait time for surgery is four weeks, with 82.2% waiting less than three months.

While physician income initially boomed after the implementation of a single-payer program, a reduction in physician salaries followed, which many feared would be a long-term result of government-run healthcare. However, by the beginning of the 21st century, medical professionals were again among Canada's top earners.

Taiwan

Healthcare in Taiwan is administrated by the Department of Health of the Executive Yuan. As with other developed economies, Taiwanese people are well-nourished but face such health problems as chronic obesity and heart disease. In 2002, Taiwan had nearly 1.6 physicians and 5.9 hospital beds per 1,000 population. In 2002, there were a total of 36 hospitals and 2,601 clinics in the country. Per capita health expenditures totaled US$752 in 2000. Health expenditures constituted 5.8 percent of the gross domestic product (GDP) in 2001 (or US$951 in 2009); 64.9 percent of the expenditures were from public funds. Despite the initial shock on Taiwan's economy from increased costs of expanded healthcare coverage, the single-payer system has provided protection from greater financial risks and has made healthcare more financially accessible for the population, resulting in a steady 70% public satisfaction rating.

The current healthcare system in Taiwan, known as National Health Insurance (NHI), was instituted in 1995. NHI is a single-payer compulsory social insurance plan which centralizes the disbursement of health care funds. The system promises equal access to health care for all citizens, and the population coverage had reached 99% by the end of 2004. NHI is mainly financed through premiums, which are based on the payroll tax, and is supplemented with out-of-pocket payments and direct government funding. In the initial stage, fee-for-service predominated for both public and private providers. Most health providers operate in the private sector and form a competitive market on the health delivery side. However, many healthcare providers took advantage of the system by offering unnecessary services to a larger number of patients and then billing the government. In the face of increasing loss and the need for cost containment, NHI changed the payment system from fee-for-service to a global budget, a kind of prospective payment system, in 2002. Taiwan's success with a single-payer health insurance program is owed, in part, to the country's human resources and the government's organizational skills, allowing for the effective and efficient management of the government-run health insurance program.

Countries with Hybrid single-payer/private Insurance Systems

Australia

Healthcare in Australia is provided by both private and government institutions. Medicare is the publicly funded universal health care venture in Australia. It was instituted in 1984 and coexists with a private health system. Medicare is funded partly by a 2% income tax levy (with exceptions for low-income earners), but mostly out of general revenue. An additional levy of 1% is imposed on high-income earners without private health insurance. As well as Medicare, there is a separate Pharmaceutical Benefits Scheme that considerably subsidises a range of prescription medications. The Minister for Health administers national health policy, elements of which (such as the operation of hospitals) are overseen by individual states.

France

Every active legal resident in France benefits from a national health insurance scheme called "Sécurité sociale". It covers 70% of the cost for all medical interventions (80% in hospitals) and tests, consultations, prescription drugs and medical devices . Pregnancy and long-time affection diseases are completely covered. Medications recognized as irreplaceable and costly are reimbursed by 100%, and less according to their necessity with a pro-rata of 65, 30 or 15% . The CPAM is also the fund for Children's mental and physical handicap institutions and invalidity . The social security is accessible to the partner and child(ren) of the beneficient. In the region of Alsace-Moselle, because of the "Concordat", the social security covers 90% of medical costs.

People legally living on the territory have access to a national health insurance known as "Couverture Maladie Universelle", which can also to some restraints deliver a complementary.

Illegals residents under a certain limit of income have access to some help called "Aide Médicale d'Etat", which is valid for 1 year and can be reconducted. Children in this condition have normal reimboursment.

To complement the remaining 30% and the additionnal eventual additionnal fees asked by hospitals and doctors, 90% of France's residents have a private, supplemental insurance, known as a "complémentaire santé", which is either provided by their employer or purchased on the market.

Spain

Building upon less structured foundations, in 1963 the existence of a single-payer healthcare system in Spain was established by the Spanish government. The system was sustained by contributions from workers, and covered them and their dependants. The universality of the system was established later in 1986. At the same time, management of public healthcare was delegated to the different autonomous communities in the country.

While previously this was not the case, in 1997 it was established that public authorities can delegate management of publicly funded healthcare to private companies. Additionally, in parallel to the single-payer healthcare system there are private insurers, which provide coverage for some private doctors and hospitals. Employers will sometimes offer private health insurance as a benefit, with 14.8% of the Spanish population being covered under private health insurance in 2013.

In 2000, the Spanish healthcare system was rated by the World Health Organization as the 7th best in the world.

United Kingdom

Healthcare in the United Kingdom is a devolved matter, meaning England, Northern Ireland, Scotland and Wales each have their own systems of private and publicly funded healthcare, generally referred to as the National Health Service (NHS). Each country having different policies and priorities has resulted in a variety of differences existing between the systems. That said, each country provides public healthcare to all UK permanent residents that is free at the point of use, being paid for from general taxation. In addition, each also has a private sector which is considerably smaller than its public equivalent, with provision of private healthcare acquired by means of private health insurance, funded as part of an employer funded healthcare scheme or paid directly by the customer, though provision can be restricted for those with conditions such as AIDS/HIV.

The individual systems are:

- England: National Health Service

- Northern Ireland: Health and Social Care in Northern Ireland (HSCNI)

- Scotland: NHS Scotland

- Wales: NHS Wales

In England, funding from general taxation is channeled through NHS England, which is responsible for commissioning mainly specialist services and primary care, and Clinical Commissioning Groups (CCGs), which hold 60% of the budget and are responsible for commissioning health services for their local populations. These commissioning bodies do not provide services themselves directly, but procure these from NHS Trusts and Foundation Trusts, as well as private, voluntary and social enterprise sector providers.

United States

Medicare in the United States is a single-payer healthcare system, but is restricted to persons over the age of 65, people under 65 who have specific disabilities, and anyone with End-Stage Renal Disease. A number of proposals have been made for a universal single-payer healthcare system in the United States, most recently the United States National Health Care Act, (popularly known as H.R. 676 or "Medicare for All," introduced in the House in February 2015) but none has achieved more than 20% congressional co-sponsorship.

Advocates argue that preventive healthcare expenditures can save several hundreds of billions of dollars per year because publicly funded universal healthcare would benefit employers and consumers, that employers would benefit from a bigger pool of potential customers and that employers would likely pay less, would be spared administrative costs, and inequities between employers would be reduced. Advocates also argue that single-payer could benefit from a more fluid economy with increasing economic growth, aggregate demand, corporate profit, and quality of life. Also, for example, cancer patients are more likely to be diagnosed at Stage I where curative treatment is typically a few outpatient visits, instead of at Stage III or later in an emergency room where treatment can involve years of hospitalization and is often terminal. Others have estimated a long-term savings amounting to 40% of all national health expenditures due to preventive health care, although estimates from the Congressional Budget Office and *The New England Journal of Medicine* have found that preventive care is more expensive due to increased utilization.

Any national system would be paid for in part through taxes replacing insurance premiums, but advocates also believe savings would be realized through preventive care and the elimination of insurance company overhead and hospital billing costs. A 2008 analysis of a single-payer bill by Physicians for a National Health Program estimated the immediate savings at $350 billion per year. The Commonwealth Fund believes that, if the United States adopted a universal health care system, the mortality rate would improve and the country would save approximately $570 billion a year.

Opponents argue single-payer does not translate into better health care. Instead, access to health care diminishes under single-payer systems, and the overall quality of care suffers. Opponents also claim that single-payer systems cause shortages of general physicians and specialists and reduce access to medical technology. As an example, Heartland Institute Senior Fellow Peter Ferrara has claimed only one-quarter of women in the United States diagnosed with breast cancer die of it, whereas the corresponding death rates are 35 percent in France and 46 percent in Britain, two nations with single-payer health-care systems. Stephen Halls, a Canadian radiologist and breast cancer researcher, however, has noted that "[s]tatistics for breast cancer incidence and mortality rates for ten year intervals in Canada, do not differ significantly from breast cancer incidence and mortality rates in the United States." Given that Canada is the United States's closest neighbor with a single payer system, it is unclear why Ferrara omitted Canada from his analysis.

National Policies and Proposals

Government is increasingly involved in U.S. health care spending, paying about 45% of the $2.2 trillion the nation spent on individuals' medical care in 2004. However, studies have shown that the publicly administered share of health spending in the U.S. may be closer to 60% as of 2002. According to Princeton University health economist Uwe Reinhardt, U.S. Medicare, Medicaid, and State Children's Health Insurance Program (SCHIP) represent "forms of 'social insurance' coupled with a largely private health-care delivery system" rather than forms of "socialized medicine." In contrast, he describes the Veterans Administration healthcare system as a pure form of socialized medicine because it is "owned, operated and financed by government."

In a peer-reviewed paper published in the *Annals of Internal Medicine*, researchers of the RAND Corporation reported that the quality of care received by Veterans Administration patients scored significantly higher overall than did comparable metrics for patients currently using United States Medicare.

The United States National Health Care Act is a perennial piece of legislation introduced in the United States House of Representatives by Representative John Conyers (D-MI) every year since 2002. The act would establish a universal single-payer health care system in the United States, the rough equivalent of Canada's Medicare, the United Kingdom's National Health Service, and Taiwan's Bureau of National Health Insurance, among other examples. Under a single-payer system, all medical care would be paid for by the Government of the United States, ending the need for private health insurance and premiums, and probably recasting private insurance companies as providing purely supplemental coverage, to be used when non-essential care is sought. The bill was first introduced in 2002, and has been reintroduced in each Congress since. During the 2009 health care debates over the bill that became the Patient Protection and Affordable Care Act, H.R. 676 was expected to be debated and voted upon by the House in September 2009, but was never debated.

The Congressional Budget Office and related government agencies scored the cost of a single-payer health care system several times since 1991. The General Accounting Office published a report in 1991 noting that "[I]f the US were to shift to a system of universal coverage and a single payer, as in Canada, the savings in administrative costs [10 percent of health spending] would be more than enough to offset the expense of universal coverage." The CBO scored the cost in 1991, noting that "the population that is currently uninsured could be covered without dramatically increasing national spending on health" and that "all US residents might be covered by health insurance for roughly the current level of spending or even somewhat less, because of savings in administrative costs and lower payment rates for services used by the privately insured." A CBO report in 1993 stated that "[t]he net cost of achieving universal insurance coverage under this single payer system would be negative" in part because "consumer payments for health would fall by $1,118 per capita, but taxes would have to increase by $1,261 per capita" in order to pay for the plan. A July 1993 scoring also resulted in positive outcomes, with the CBO stating that, "[a]s the program was phased in, the administrative savings from switching to a single-payer system would offset much of the increased demand for health care services. Later, the cap on the growth of the national health budget would hold the rate of growth of spending below the baseline." The CBO also scored Sen. Paul Wellstone's American Health and Security Act of 1993 in December 1993, finding that "by year five (and in subsequent years) the new system would cost less than baseline." A 2014 study published in the journal BMC Medical Services Research by James Kahn, et al., found that the actual administrative burden of health care in the United States was 27% of all national health expenditures. The study examined both direct costs charged by insurers for profit, administration and marketing but also the indirect burden placed on health care providers like hospitals, nursing homes and doctors for costs they incurred in working with private health insurers including contract negotiations, financial and clinical record-keeping (variable and idiosyncratic for each payer). Kahn, et al. estimate that the added cost for the private insurer health system in the US was about $471 billion in 2012 compared to a single-payer system like Canada's. This represents just over 20% of the total national healthcare expenditure in 2012. Kahn asserts that this excess administrative cost will increase under the Affordable Care Act with its reliance on the provision of health coverage through a multi-payer system.

State Proposals

Several single-payer state referendums and bills from state legislatures have been proposed, but, with the exception of Vermont, all have failed. In December 2014, Vermont canceled its plan for single-payer health care.

California

California attempted passage of a single-payer bill as early as 1994, and the first successful passages of legislation through the California State Legislature, SB 840 or "The California Universal Healthcare Act" (authored by Sheila Kuehl), occurred in 2006 and again in 2008. Both times, Governor Arnold Schwarzenegger vetoed the bill. State Senator Mark Leno has reintroduced the bill in each legislative session since. In June 2017 the California State Senate passed a single-payer bill initiated by State Senator Ricardo Lara.

Colorado

The Colorado State Health Care System Initiative, Amendment 69, was a citizen-initiated constitutional amendment proposal in November 2016 to vote on a single-payer healthcare system funded by a 10% payroll tax split 2:1 between employers and employees. This would have replaced the private health insurance premiums currently paid by employees and companies. The ballot was rejected by 79% of the electorate.

Hawaii

In 2009, the Hawaii state legislature passed a single-payer healthcare bill that was vetoed by Republican Governor Linda Lingle. While the veto was overridden by the legislature, the bill was not implemented.

Illinois

In 2007, the Health Care for All Illinois Act was introduced and the Illinois House of Representatives' Health Availability Access Committee passed the single-payer bill favorably out of committee by an 8–4 vote. The legislation was eventually referred back to the House rules committee and not taken up again during that session.

Massachusetts

Massachusetts had passed a universal healthcare program in 1986, but budget constraints and partisan control of the legislature resulted in its repeal before the legislation could be enacted. Question 4, a nonbinding referendum, was on the ballot in 14 state districts in November 2010, asking voters, "[S]hall the representative from this district be instructed to support legislation that would establish healthcare as a human right regardless of age, state of health or employment status, by creating a single payer health insurance system like Medicare that is comprehensive, cost effective, and publicly provided to all residents of Massachusetts?" The ballot question passed in all 14 districts that offered the question.

Minnesota

The Minnesota Health Act, which would establish a statewide single-payer health plan, has been presented to the Minnesota legislature regularly since 2009. The bill was passed out of both the Senate Health Housing and Family Security Committee and the Senate Commerce and Consumer Protection Committee in 2009, but the House version was ultimately tabled. In 2010, the bill passed the Senate Judiciary Committee on a voice vote as well as the House Health Care & Human Services Policy and Oversight Committee. In 2011, the bill was introduced as a two-year bill in both the Senate and House, but did not progress. It has been introduced again in the 2013 session in both chambers.

Montana

In September 2011, Governor Brian Schweitzer announced his intention to seek a waiver from the federal government allowing Montana to set up a single-payer healthcare system. Governor Schweitzer was unable to implement single-payer health care in Montana, but did make moves to open government-run clinics and, in his final budget as governor, increased coverage for lower-income Montana residents.

New York

New York State has been attempting passage of the New York Health Act, which would establish a statewide single-payer health plan, since 1992. The New York Health Act passed the Assembly four times: once in 1992 and again in 2015, 2016, and 2017, but has not yet advanced through the Senate after referrals to the Health Committee. On all occasions, the legislation passed the Assembly by an almost two-to-one ratio of support.

Oregon

The state of Oregon attempted to pass single-payer healthcare via Oregon Ballot Measure 23 in 2002, and the measure was rejected by a significant majority. Previous bills, including the Affordable Health Care for All Oregon Act, have been introduced in the legislature but have never left committee.

Pennsylvania

The Family Business and Healthcare Security Act has been introduced in the Pennsylvania legislature numerous times, but has never been able to pass.

Vermont

In December 2014, Vermont canceled its plan for single-payer healthcare. Vermont passed legislation in 2011 creating Green Mountain Care. When Governor Peter Shumlin signed the bill into law, Vermont became the first state to functionally have a single-payer health care system. While the bill is considered a single-payer bill, private insurers can continue to operate in the state indefinitely, meaning it does not fit the strict definition of single-payer. Representative Mark Larson, the initial sponsor of the bill, has described Green Mountain Care's provisions "as close as we can get [to single-payer] at the state level."

Vermont abandoned the plan in 2014, citing costs and tax increases as too high to implement.

Public Opinion

Advocates for single-payer point to support in polls, although the polling is mixed depending on how the question is asked. Polls from Harvard University in 1988, the Los Angeles Times in 1990, and the Wall Street Journal in 1991 all showed strong support for a health care system comparable to the system in Canada. More recently, however, polling support has declined. A 2007 Yahoo/AP poll showed a majority of respondents considered themselves supporters of "single-payer health care," and a plurality of respondents in a 2009 poll for Time Magazine showed support for "a national single-payer plan similar to Medicare for all." Polls by Rasmussen Reports in 2011 and 2012 showed pluralities opposed to single-payer health care.

A 2001 article in the public health journal *Health Affairs* studied fifty years of American public opinion of various health care plans and concluded that, while there appears to be general support of a "national health care plan," poll respondents "remain satisfied with their current medical arrangements, do not trust the federal government to do what is right, and do not favor a single-payer type of national health plan." Politifact rated a statement by Michael Moore "false" when he stated that "[t]he majority actually want single-payer health care." According to Politifact, responses on these polls largely depend on the wording. For example, people respond more favorably when they are asked if they want a system "like Medicare."

Advocacy Groups

Physicians for a National Health Program the American Medical Student Association, Health-care-NOW! and the California Nurses Association are among advocacy groups that have called for the introduction of a single-payer healthcare program in the United States. A 2007 study published in the *Annals of Internal Medicine* found that 59% of physicians "supported legislation to establish national health insurance" while 9% were neutral on the topic, and 32% opposed it.

Universal Health Care

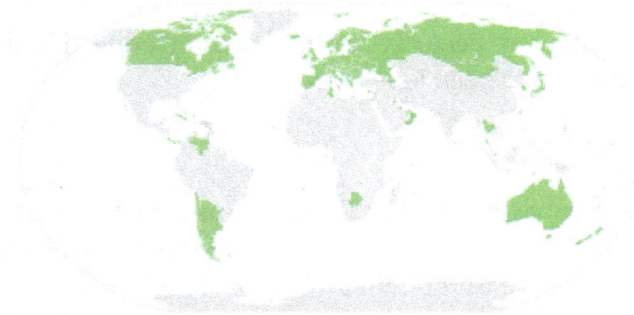

As of 2009, 58 countries have legislation mandating universal health care and have actually reached >90% health insurance coverage and >90% skilled birth attendance.

Universal health care, sometimes referred to as universal health coverage, universal coverage, or universal care, usually refers to a health care system that provides health care and financial protection to all citizens of a particular country. It is organized around providing a specified package of benefits to all members of a society with the end goal of providing financial risk protection, improved access to health services, and improved health outcomes. Universal health care is not one-size-fits-all and does not imply coverage for all people for everything. Universal health care can be determined by three critical dimensions: who is covered, what services are covered, and how much of the cost is covered. It is described by the World Health Organization as a situation where citizens can access health services without incurring financial hardship. U.N. member states have agreed to work toward universal health coverage by 2030.

History

The first move towards a national health insurance system was launched in Germany in 1883, with the Sickness Insurance Law. Industrial employers were mandated to provide injury and illness insurance for their low-wage workers, and the system was funded and administered by employees and employers through "sick funds", which were drawn from deductions in workers' wages and from employers' contributions. Other countries soon began to follow suit. In the United Kingdom, the National Insurance Act 1911 provided coverage for primary care (but not specialist or hospital care) for wage earners, covering about one third of the population. The Russian Empire established a similar system in 1912, and other industrialized countries began following suit. By the 1930s, similar systems existed in virtually all of Western and Central Europe. Japan introduced an employee health insurance law in 1927, expanding further upon it in 1935 and 1940. Following the Russian Revolution of 1917, the Soviet Union established a fully public and centralized health care system in 1920. However, it was not a truly universal system at that point, as rural residents were not covered.

In New Zealand, a universal health care system was created in a series of steps, from 1939 to 1941. In Australia, the state of Queensland introduced a free public hospital system in the 1940s.

Following World War II, universal health care systems began to be set up around the world. On July 5, 1948, the United Kingdom launched its universal National Health Service. Universal health care was next introduced in the Nordic countries of Sweden (1955), Iceland (1956), Norway (1956), Denmark (1961), and Finland (1964). Universal health insurance was then introduced in Japan (1961), and in Canada through stages, starting with the province of Saskatchewan in 1962, followed by the rest of Canada from 1968 to 1972. The Soviet Union extended universal health care to its rural residents in 1969. Italy introduced its *Servizio Sanitario Nazionale* (National Health Service) in 1978. Universal health insurance was implemented in Australia beginning with the *Medibank* system in 1975, which led to universal coverage under the Medicare system, established in 1984.

From the 1970s to the 2000s, Southern and Western European countries began introducing universal coverage, most of them building upon previous health insurance programs to cover the whole population. For example, France built upon its 1928 national health insurance system, with subsequent legislation covering a larger and larger percentage of the population, until the remaining 1% of the population that was uninsured received coverage in 2000. In addition, universal health coverage was introduced in some Asian countries, including South Korea (1989), Taiwan (1995), Israel (1995), and Thailand (2001).

Following the collapse of the Soviet Union, Russia retained and reformed its universal health care system, as did other former Soviet nations and Eastern bloc countries.

Beyond the 1990s, many countries in Latin America, the Caribbean, Africa, and the Asia-Pacific region, including developing countries, took steps to bring their populations under universal health coverage, including China which has the largest universal health care system in the world. A 2012 study examined progress being made by these countries, focusing on nine in particular: Ghana, Rwanda, Nigeria, Mali, Kenya, India, Indonesia, the Philippines, and Vietnam.

Funding Models

Universal health care in most countries has been achieved by a mixed model of funding. General taxation revenue is the primary source of funding, but in many countries it is supplemented by specific levies (which may be charged to the individual and/or an employer) or with the option of private payments (by direct or optional insurance) for services beyond those covered by the public system.

Almost all European systems are financed through a mix of public and private contributions. Most universal health care systems are funded primarily by tax revenue (like in Portugal Spain, Denmark, and Sweden). Some nations, such as Germany and France and Japan employ a multipayer system in which health care is funded by private and public contributions. However, much of the non-government funding is by contributions by employers and employees to regulated non-profit sickness funds. Contributions are compulsory and defined according to law.

A distinction is also made between municipal and national healthcare funding. For example, one model is that the bulk of the healthcare is funded by the municipality, speciality healthcare is provided and possibly funded by a larger entity, such as a municipal co-operation board or the state, and the medications are paid by a state agency.

Universal health care systems are modestly redistributive. The progressivity of health care financing has limited implications for overall income inequality.

Compulsory Insurance

This is usually enforced via legislation requiring residents to purchase insurance, but sometimes the government provides the insurance. Sometimes, there may be a choice of multiple public and private funds providing a standard service (as in Germany) or sometimes just a single public fund (as in Canada). Healthcare in Switzerland and the US Patient Protection and Affordable Care Act are based on compulsory insurance.

In some European countries in which private insurance and universal health care coexist, such as Germany, Belgium, and the Netherlands, the problem of adverse selection is overcome by using a risk compensation pool to equalize, as far as possible, the risks between funds. Thus, a fund with a predominantly healthy, younger population has to pay into a compensation pool and a fund with an older and predominantly less healthy population would receive funds from the pool. In this way, sickness funds compete on price, and there is no advantage to eliminate people with higher risks because they are compensated for by means of risk-adjusted capitation payments. Funds are not allowed to pick and choose their policyholders or deny coverage, but they compete mainly on price and service. In some countries, the basic coverage level is set by the government and cannot be modified.

The Republic of Ireland at one time had a "community rating" system by VHI, effectively a single-payer or common risk pool. The government later opened VHI to competition but without a compensation pool. That resulted in foreign insurance companies entering the Irish market and offering cheap health insurance to relatively healthy segments of the market, which then made higher profits at VHI's expense. The government later reintroduced community rating by a pooling arrangement and at least one main major insurance company, BUPA, then withdrew from the Irish market.

Among the potential solutions posited by economists are single-payer systems as well as other methods of ensuring that health insurance is universal, such as by requiring all citizens to purchase insurance or limiting the ability of insurance companies to deny insurance to individuals or vary price between individuals.

Single Payer

Single-payer health care is a system in which the government, rather than private insurers, pays for all health care costs. Single-payer systems may contract for healthcare services from private organizations (as is the case in Canada) or own and employ healthcare resources and personnel (as was the case in England before of the Health and Social Care Act). "Single-payer" thus describes only the funding mechanism and refers to health care financed by a single public body from a single fund and does not specify the type of delivery or for whom doctors work. Although the fund holder is usually the state, some forms of single-payer use a mixed public-private system.

Tax-based Financing

In tax-based financing, individuals contribute to the provision of health services through various taxes. These are typically pooled across the whole population, unless local governments raise and retain tax revenues. Some countries (notably the United Kingdom, Canada, Ireland, Australia, New Zealand, Italy, Spain, Portugal and the Nordic countries) choose to fund health care directly from taxation alone. Other countries with insurance-based systems effectively meet the cost of insuring those unable to insure themselves via social security arrangements funded from taxation, either by directly paying their medical bills or by paying for insurance premiums for those affected.

Social Health Insurance

In social health insurance, contributions from workers, the self-employed, enterprises and government are pooled into a single or multiple funds on a compulsory basis. The funds typically contract with a mix of public and private providers for the provision of a specified benefit package. Preventive and public health care may be provided by these funds or responsibility kept solely by the Ministry of Health. Within social health insurance, a number of functions may be executed by parastatal or non-governmental sickness funds or in a few cases by private health insurance companies.

Private Insurance

In private health insurance, premiums are paid directly from employers, associations, individuals and families to insurance companies, which pool risks across their membership base. Private insurance includes policies sold by commercial for profit firms, non-profit companies, and community health insurers. Generally, private insurance is voluntary in contrast to social insurance programs, which tend to be compulsory.

In some countries with universal coverage, private insurance often excludes many health conditions that are expensive and the state health care system can provide. For example, in the United Kingdom, one of the largest private health care providers is BUPA, which has a long list of general exclusions even in its highest coverage policy, most of which are routinely provided by the National Health Service. In the United States, dialysis treatment for end stage renal failure is generally paid for by government, not by the insurance industry. Those with privatized Medicare (Medicare Advantage) are the exception and must get their dialysis paid through their insurance company, but those with end stage renal failure generally cannot buy Medicare Advantage plans.

The Planning Commission of India has also suggested that the country should embrace insurance to achieve universal health coverage. General tax revenue is currently used to meet the essential health requirements of all people.

Community-based Health Insurance

A particular form of private health insurance that has often emerged if financial risk protection mechanisms have only a limited impact is community-based health insurance. Individual members of a specific community pay to a collective health fund, which they can draw from when they need of medical care. Contributions are not risk-related, and there is generally a high level of community involvement in the running of these plans.

Implementation and Comparisons

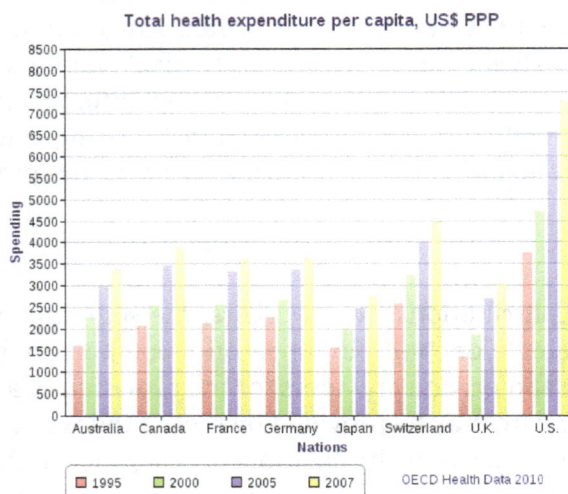

Total health expenditure per capita, US$ PPP

1995   2000   2005   2007   OECD Health Data 2010

Health spending per capita, in US$ purchasing power parity-adjusted, among various OECD countries

Universal health care systems vary according to the degree of government involvement in providing care and/or health insurance. In some countries, such as the UK, Spain, Italy, Australia and the Nordic countries, the government has a high degree of involvement in the commissioning or delivery of health care services and access is based on residence rights, not on the purchase of insurance. Others have a much more pluralistic delivery system, based on obligatory health with contributory insurance rates related to salaries or income and usually funded by employers and beneficiaries jointly.

Sometimes, the health funds are derived from a mixture of insurance premiums, salary related mandatory contributions by employees and/or employers to regulated sickness funds, and by government taxes. These insurance based systems tend to reimburse private or public medical providers, often at heavily regulated rates, through mutual or publicly owned medical insurers. A few countries, such as the Netherlands and Switzerland, operate via privately owned but heavily regulated private insurers, which are not allowed to make a profit from the mandatory element of insurance but can profit by selling supplemental insurance.

Universal health care is a broad concept that has been implemented in several ways. The common denominator for all such programs is some form of government action aimed at extending access to health care as widely as possible and setting minimum standards. Most implement universal health care through legislation, regulation and taxation. Legislation and regulation direct what care must be provided, to whom, and on what basis. Usually, some costs are borne by the patient at the time of consumption, but the bulk of costs come from a combination of compulsory insurance and tax revenues. Some programs are paid for entirely out of tax revenues. In others, tax revenues are used either to fund insurance for the very poor or for those needing long-term chronic care.

The United Kingdom National Audit Office in 2003 published an international comparison of ten different health care systems in ten developed countries, nine universal systems against one non-universal system (the United States), and their relative costs and key health outcomes. A wider international comparison of 16 countries, each with universal health care, was published by the World Health Organization in 2004. In some cases, government involvement also includes directly managing the health care system, but many countries use mixed public-private systems to deliver universal health care.

Health Informatics

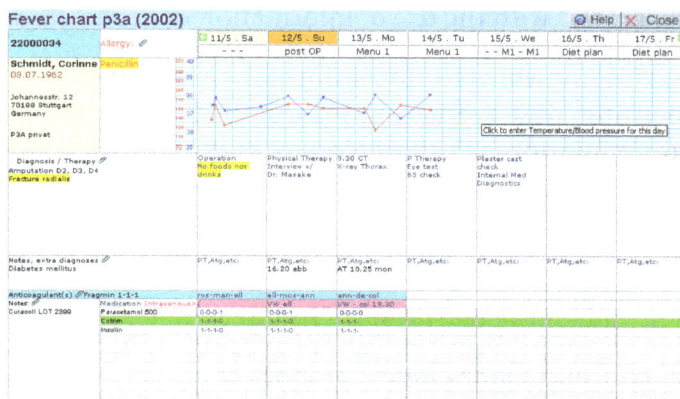

Electronic patient chart from a health information system

Health informatics (also called health care informatics, healthcare informatics, medical informatics, nursing informatics, clinical informatics, or biomedical informatics) is informatics in health care. It is a multidisciplinary field that uses health information technology (HIT) to improve health care via any combination of higher quality, higher efficiency (spurring lower cost and thus greater availability), and new opportunities. The disciplines involved include information science, computer science, social science, behavioral science, management science, and others. The NLM defines health informatics as "the interdisciplinary study of the design, development, adoption and application of IT-based innovations in healthcare services delivery, management and planning." It deals with the resources, devices, and methods required to optimize the acquisition, storage, retrieval, and use of information in health and biomedicine. Health informatics tools include amongst others computers, clinical guidelines, formal medical terminologies, and information and communication systems. It is applied to the areas of nursing, clinical medicine, dentistry, pharmacy, public health, occupational therapy, physical therapy, biomedical research, and alternative medicine. All of which are designed to improve the overall of effectiveness of patient care delivery by ensuring that the data generated is of a high quality e.g. an mHealth based early warning scorecard.

- The international standards on the subject are covered by ICS 35.240.80 in which ISO 27799:2008 is one of the core components.

- Molecular bioinformatics and clinical informatics have converged into the field of translational bioinformatics.

Sub Specialities

Healthcare informatics includes the subspecialties of clinical informatics, pathology informatics, imaging informatics, and pharmacy informatics

It also includes public health informatics, community health informatics, home health informatics, nursing informatics, medical informatics, consumer health informatics, clinical bioinformatics, and informatics for education and research in health and medicine.

Healthcare Informatics

Clinical Informatics

Clinical informatics is concerned with the use of information in health care by and for clinicians.

Clinical informaticians, also known as clinical informaticists, transform health care by analyzing, designing, implementing, and evaluating information and communication systems that enhance individual and population health outcomes, improve [patient] care, and strengthen the clinician-patient relationship. Clinical informaticians use their knowledge of patient care combined with their understanding of informatics concepts, methods, and health informatics tools to:

- assess information and knowledge needs of health care professionals and patients,

- characterize, evaluate, and refine clinical processes,

- develop, implement, and refine clinical decision support systems, and

- lead or participate in the procurement, customization, development, implementation, management, evaluation, and continuous improvement of clinical information systems.

Clinicians collaborate with other health care and information technology professionals to develop health informatics tools which promote patient care that is safe, efficient, effective, timely, patient-centered, and equitable. Many clinical informaticists are also computer scientists.

In October 2011 American Board of Medical Specialties (ABMS), the organization overseeing the certification of specialist MDs in the United States, announced the creation of MD-only physician certification in clinical informatics. The first examination for board certification in the subspecialty of clinical informatics was offered in October 2013 by American Board of Preventive Medicine (ABPM) with 432 passing to become the 2014 inaugural class of Diplomates in clinical informatics.

Fellowship programs exist for physicians who wish to become board-certified in clinical informatics. Physicians must have graduated from a medical school in the United States or Canada, or a school located elsewhere that is approved by the ABPM. In addition, they must complete a primary residency program such as Internal Medicine (or any of the 24 subspecialties recognized by the ABMS) and be eligible to become licensed to practice medicine in the state where their fellowship program is located. The fellowship program is 24 months in length, with fellows dividing their time between Informatics rotations, didactics, research, and clinical work in their primary specialty.

Integrated Data Repository

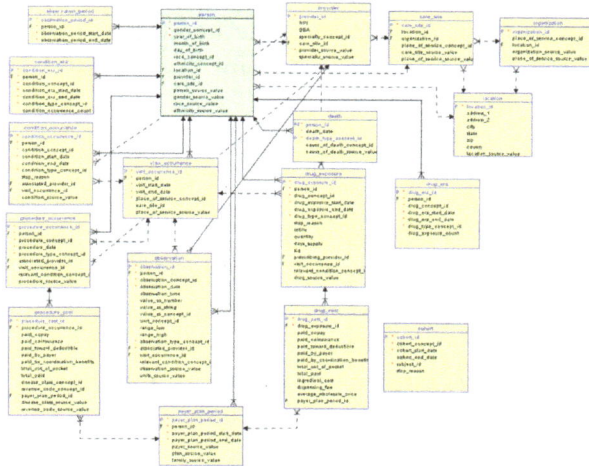

example IDR schema

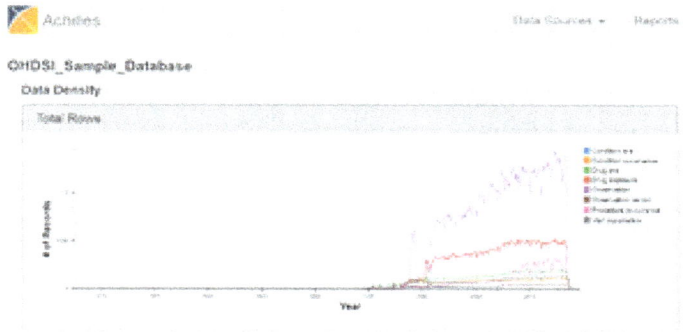

Achilles tool for data characterization of a healthcare dataset

One of the fundamental elements of biomedical and translational research is the use of integrated data repositories. Survey conducted in 2010, defined "integrated data repository" (IDR) as a data warehouse incorporating various sources of clinical data to support queries for a range of research-like functions. Integrated data repositories are complex systems developed to solve a variety of problems ranging from identity management, protection of confidentiality, semantic and syntactic comparability of data from different sources, and most importantly convenient and flexible query. Development of the field of clinical informatics lead to the creation of large data sets with electronic health record data integrated with other data (such as genomic data). Types of data repositories include operational data stores (ODSs), clinical data warehouses, clinical data marts, and clinical registries. Operational data stores established for extracting, transferring and loading before creating warehouse or data marts. Clinical registries repositories have long been in existence, but their contents are disease specific and sometimes considered archaic. Clinical data stores and clinical data warehouses are considered fast and reliable. Though these large integrated repositories have impacted clinical research significantly, it still faces challenges and barriers. One big problem is the requirement for ethical approval by the institutional review board (IRB) for each research analysis meant for publication. Some research resources do not require individual IRB approval, example CDWs with data of deceased patients have been de-identified, and its usage does not require institutional review board (IRB) approval. However, privacy sensitive data may still be explored by researchers when shared through its metadata and services, for example by following a linked open data perspective. Another challenge is data quality. Methods that adjust for bias (such as using propensity score matching methods) assume that complete health record is captured. Tools that examine data quality (e.g., point to missing data) help in discovering data quality problems.

Clinical Research Informatics

Clinical research informatics (CRI) is a subfield of health informatics that tries to improve the efficiency of clinical research by using informatics methods. Some of the problems tackled by CRI are: creation of data warehouses of healthcare data that can be used for research, support of data collection in clinical trials by the use of electronic data capture systems, streamlining ethical approvals and renewals (in US the responsible entity is the local institutional review board), maintenance of repositories of past clinical trial data (de-identified).

CRI is a fairly new branch of informatics and has met growing pains as any up and coming field does. Some issues CRI faces is the ability for the statisticians and the computer system architects to work with the clinical research staff in designing a system and lack of funding to support the development of a new system. Researchers and the informatics team have a difficult time coordinating plans and ideas in order to design a system that is easy to use for the research team yet fits in the system requirements of the computer team. The lack of funding can be a hindrance to the development of the CRI. Many organizations who are performing research are struggling to get financial support to conduct the research, much less invest that money in an informatics system that will not provide them any more income or improve the outcome of the research (Embi, 2009).

Common Data Elements (CDEs) in Clinical Research

Ability to integrate data from multiple clinical trials is an important part of clinical research informatics. Initiatives, such as PhenX and Patient-Reported Outcomes Measurement Information System triggered a general effort to improve secondary use of data collected in past human clinical trials. CDE initiatives, for example, try to allow clinical trial designers to adopt standardized research instruments (electronic case report forms).

Human Bioinformatics

Translational Bioinformatics

With the completion of the human genome and the recent advent of high throughput sequencing and genome-wide association studies of single nucleotide polymorphisms, the fields of molecular bioinformatics, biostatistics, statistical genetics and clinical informatics are converging into the emerging field of translational bioinformatics.

The relationship between bioinformatics and health informatics, while conceptually related under the umbrella of biomedical informatics, has not always been very clear. The TBI community is specifically motivated with the development of approaches to identify linkages between fundamental biological and clinical information.

Along with complementary areas of emphasis, such as those focused on developing systems and approaches within clinical research contexts, insights from TBI may enable a new paradigm for the study and treatment of disease.

Translational Bioinformatics (TBI) is a relatively new field that surfaced in the year of 2000 when human genome sequence was released (Tenenbaum, 2016). The commonly used definition of TBI is lengthy and could be found on the. In simpler terms, TBI could be defined as a collection of colossal amounts of health related data (biomedical and genomic) and translation of the data into individually tailored clinical entities (Tenenbaum, 2016). Today, TBI field is categorized into four major themes that are briefly described below:

1. Clinical big data

    Clinical big data is a collection of electronic health records that are used for innovations. The evidence-based approach that is currently practiced in medicine is suggested to be merged with the practice-based medicine to achieve better outcomes for patients. As CEO of California-based cognitive computing firm Apixio, Darren Schutle, explains that the care can be better fitted to the patient if the data could be collected from various medical records, merged, and analyzed. Further, the combination of similar profiles can serve as a basis for personalized medicine pointing to what works and what does not for certain condition (Marr, 2016).

2. Genomics in clinical care

    Genomic data are used to identify the genes involvement in unknown or rare conditions/syndromes. Currently, the most vigorous area of using genomics is oncology. The identification of genomic sequencing of cancer may define reasons of drug(s) sensitivity and resistance during oncological treatment processes (Tenenbaum, 2016).

3. Omics for drugs discovery and repurposing

    The drug repurposing is an appealing idea that allows the pharmaceutical companies to sell an already approved drug to treat a different condition/disease that the drug was not initially approved for by the FDA. The observation of "molecular signatures in disease and compare those to signatures observed in cells" points to the possibility of a drug ability to cure and/or relieve symptoms of a disease (Tenenbaum, 2016).

4. Personalized genomic testing

    In the USA, several companies offer direct-to-consumer (DTC) genetic testing. The company that performs the majority of testing is called 23andMe. Utilizing genetic testing in health care raises many ethical, legal and social concerns; one of the main questions is whether the healthcare providers are ready to include patient-supplied genomic information while providing care that is unbiased (despite the intimate genomic knowledge) and a high quality. The documented examples of incorporating such information into a healthcare delivery showed both positive and negative impacts on the overall healthcare related outcomes (Tenenbaum, 2016).

Computational Health Informatics

Computational health informatics is a branch of computer science that deals specifically with computational techniques that are relevant in healthcare. Computational health informatics is also a branch of health informatics, but is orthogonal to much of the work going on in health informatics because computer scientist's interest is mainly in understanding fundamental properties of computation. Health informatics, on the other hand, is primarily concerned with understanding fundamental properties of medicine that allow for the intervention of computers. The health domain provides an extremely wide variety of problems that can be tackled using computational techniques, and computer scientists are attempting to make a difference in medicine by studying the underlying principles of computer science that will allow for meaningful (to medicine) algorithms and systems to be developed. Thus, computer scientists working in computational health informatics and health scientists working in medical health informatics combine to develop the next generation of healthcare technologies.

Using computers to analyze health data has been around since the 1950s, but it wasn't until the 1990s that the first sturdy models appeared. The development of the internet has helped develop computational health informatics over the past decade. Computer models are used to examine various topics such as how exercise affects obesity, healthcare costs, and many more.

Examples of projects in computational health informatics include the COACH project.

Informatics for Education and Research in Health and Medicine

Clinical Research Informatics

Clinical research informatics (CRI) is an amalgamation of clinical and research informatics. Featuring both clinical and research informatics, CRI has a vital role in clinical research, patient care, and the building of healthcare system (Katzan & Rudick, 2012). CRI is one of the rapidly growing subdivisions of biomedical informatics which plays an important role in developing new informatics theories, tools, and solutions to accelerate the full transitional continuum (Kahn & Weng, 2012). Evolution of CRI was extremely important in Informatics as there was an extraordinary increase in the scope and pace of clinical and translational science advancements (Katzan & Rudick, 2012). Clinical research informatics takes the core foundations, principles, and technologies related to Health Informatics, and applies these to clinical research contexts. As such, CRI is a sub-discipline of health informatics, and interest and activities in CRI have increased greatly in recent years given the overwhelming problems associated with the explosive growth of clinical research data and information. There are a number of activities within clinical research that CRI supports, including:

- more efficient and effective data collection and acquisition
- improved recruitment into clinical trials
- optimal protocol design and efficient management
- patient recruitment and management
- adverse event reporting
- regulatory compliance
- data storage, transfer, processing and analysis
- repositories of data from completed clinical trials (for secondary analyses)

History

Worldwide use of computer technology in medicine began in the early 1950s with the rise of the computers. In 1949, Gustav Wagner established the first professional organization for informatics in Germany. The prehistory, history, and future of medical information and health information technology are discussed in reference. Specialized university departments and Informatics training programs began during the 1960s in France, Germany, Belgium and The Netherlands. Medical informatics research units began to appear during the 1970s in Poland and in the U.S. Since then the development of high-quality health informatics research, education and infrastructure has been a goal of the U.S. and the European Union.

Early names for health informatics included medical computing, biomedical computing, medical computer science, computer medicine, medical electronic data processing, medical automatic data processing, medical information processing, medical information science, medical software engineering, and medical computer technology.

The health informatics community is still growing, it is by no means a mature profession, but work in the UK by the voluntary registration body, the UK Council of Health Informatics Professions has suggested eight key constituencies within the domain—information management, knowledge management, portfolio/programme/project management, ICT, education and research, clinical informatics, health records(service and business-related), health informatics service management. These constituencies accommodate professionals in and for the NHS, in academia and commercial service and solution providers.

Since the 1970s the most prominent international coordinating body has been the International Medical Informatics Association (IMIA).

In the United States

Even though the idea of using computers in medicine emerged as technology advanced in the early 20th century, it was not until the 1950s that informatics began to have an effect in the United States.

The earliest use of electronic digital computers for medicine was for dental projects in the 1950s at the United States National Bureau of Standards by Robert Ledley. During the mid-1950s, the United States Air Force (USAF) carried out several medical projects on its computers while also encouraging civilian agencies such as the National Academy of Sciences - National Research Council (NAS-NRC) and the National Institutes of Health (NIH) to sponsor such work. In 1959, Ledley and Lee B. Lusted published "Reasoning Foundations of Medical Diagnosis," a widely read article in *Science*, which introduced computing (especially operations research) techniques to medical workers. Ledley and Lusted's article has remained influential for decades, especially within the field of medical decision making.

Guided by Ledley's late 1950s survey of computer use in biology and medicine (carried out for the NAS-NRC), and by his and Lusted's articles, the NIH undertook the first major effort to introduce computers to biology and medicine. This effort, carried out initially by the NIH's Advisory Committee on Computers in Research (ACCR), chaired by Lusted, spent over $40 million between 1960 and 1964 in order to establish dozens of large and small biomedical research centers in the US.

One early (1960, non-ACCR) use of computers was to help quantify normal human movement, as a precursor to scientifically measuring deviations from normal, and design of prostheses. The use of computers (IBM 650, 1620, and 7040) allowed analysis of a large sample size, and of more measurements and subgroups than had been previously practical with mechanical calculators, thus allowing an objective understanding of how human locomotion varies by age and body characteristics. A study co-author was Dean of the Marquette University College of Engineering; this work led to discrete Biomedical Engineering departments there and elsewhere.

The next steps, in the mid-1960s, were the development (sponsored largely by the NIH) of expert systems such as MYCIN and Internist-I. In 1965, the National Library of Medicine started to use MEDLINE and MEDLARS. Around this time, Neil Pappalardo, Curtis Marble, and Robert Greenes developed MUMPS (Massachusetts General Hospital Utility Multi-Programming System) in Octo Barnett's Laboratory of Computer Science at Massachusetts General Hospital in Boston, another center of biomedical computing that received significant support from the NIH. In the 1970s and 1980s it was the most commonly used programming language for clinical applications. The MUMPS operating system was used to support MUMPS language specifications. As of 2004, a descendent of this system is being used in the United States Veterans Affairs hospital system. The VA has the largest enterprise-wide health information system that includes an electronic medical record, known as the Veterans Health Information Systems and Technology Architecture (VistA). A graphical user interface known as the Computerized Patient Record System (CPRS) allows health care providers to review and update a patient's electronic medical record at any of the VA's over 1,000 health care facilities.

During the 1960s, Morris Collen, a physician working for Kaiser Permanente's Division of Research, developed computerized systems to automate many aspects of multiphasic health checkups. These system became the basis the larger medical databases Kaiser Permanente developed during the 1970s and 1980s. The American College of Medical Informatics (ACMI) has since 1993 annually bestowed the Morris F. Collen, MD Medal for Outstanding Contributions to the Field of Medical Informatics. Kaiser permanente

In the 1970s a growing number of commercial vendors began to market practice management and electronic medical records systems. Although many products exist, only a small number of health practitioners use fully featured electronic health care records systems. In 1970, Warner Slack, MD, and Howard Bleich, MD, co-founded the academic division of clincal informatics at Beth Israel Deaconess Medical Center and Harvard Medical School. Warner Slack is a pioneer of the development of the electronic patient medical history, and in 1977 Dr. Bleich created the first user-friendly search engine for the worlds biomedical literature. In 2002, Dr. Slack and Dr. Bleich were awarded the Morris F. Collen Award for their pioneering contributions to medical informatics.

Computerized systems involved in patient care have led to a number of changes. Such changes have led to improvements in electronic health records which are now capable of sharing medical information among multiple healthcare stakeholders(Zahabi, Kaber, & Swangnetr, 2015); thereby, supporting the flow of patient information through various modalities of care.

Computer use today involves a broad ability which includes but isn't limited to physician diagnosis and documentation, patient appointment scheduling, and billing. Many researchers in the field have identified an increase in the quality of healthcare systems, decreased errors by healthcare workers, and lastly savings in time and money (Zahabi, Kaber, & Swangnetr, 2015). The system however is not perfect and will continue to require improvement. Frequently cited factors of concern involve usability, safety, accessibility, and user friendliness (Zahabi, Kaber, & Swangnetr, 2015). As leaders in the field of medical informatics improve upon the aforementioned factors of concern, the overall provision of healthcare will continue to improve.

Homer R. Warner, one of the fathers of medical informatics, founded the Department of Medical Informatics at the University of Utah in 1968. The American Medical Informatics Association (AMIA) has an award named after him on application of informatics to medicine.

Informatics Certifications

Like other IT training specialties, there are Informatics certifications available to help informatics professionals stand out and be recognized. The American Nurses Credentialing Center (ANCC) offers a board certification in Nursing Informatics. For Radiology Informatics, the CIIP (Certified Imaging Informatics Professional) certification was created by ABII (The American Board of Imaging Informatics) which was founded by SIIM (the Society for Imaging Informatics in Medicine) and ARRT (the American Registry of Radiologic Technologists) in 2005. The CIIP certification requires documented experience working in Imaging Informatics, formal testing and is a limited time credential requiring renewal every five years. The exam tests for a combination of IT technical knowledge, clinical understanding, and project management experience thought to represent the typical workload of a PACS administrator or other radiology IT clinical support role. Certifications from PARCA (PACS Administrators Registry and Certifications Association) are also recognized. The five PARCA certifications are tiered from entry level to architect level. The American Health Information Management Association offers credentials in medical coding, analytics, and data administration, such as Registered Health Information Administrator and Certified Coding Associate.

Certifications are widely requested by employers in health informatics, and overall the demand for certified informatics workers in the United States is outstripping supply. The American Health Information Management Association reports that only 68% of applicants pass certification exams on the first try.

In the UK

The broad history of health informatics has been captured in the book *UK Health Computing : Recollections and reflections*, Hayes G, Barnett D (Eds.), BCS (May 2008) by those active in the field, predominantly members of BCS Health and its constituent groups. The book describes the path taken as 'early development of health informatics was unorganized and idiosyncratic'. In the early 1950s, it was prompted by those involved in NHS finance and only in the early 1960s did solutions including those in pathology (1960), radiotherapy (1962), immunization (1963), and primary care (1968) emerge. Many of these solutions, even in the early 1970s were developed in-house by pioneers in the field to meet their own requirements. In part this was due to some areas of health services (for example the immunization and vaccination of children) still being provided by Local Authorities. Interesting, this is a situation which the coalition government propose broadly to return to in the 2010 strategy Equity and Excellence: Liberating the NHS (July 2010); stating:

"We will put patients at the heart of the NHS, through an information revolution and greater choice and control' with shared decision-making becoming the norm: 'no decision about me without me' and patients having access to the information they want, to make choices about their care. They will have increased control over their own care records."

These types of statements present a significant opportunity for health informaticians to come out of the back-office and take up a front-line role supporting clinical practice, and the business of care delivery. The UK health informatics community has long played a key role in international activity, joining TC4 of the International Federation of Information Processing (1969) which became IMIA (1979). Under the aegis of BCS Health, Cambridge was the host for the first EFMI Medical Informatics Europe (1974) conference and London was the location for IMIA's tenth global congress (MEDINFO2001).

Current State and Policy Initiatives

Argentina

Since 1997, the Buenos Aires Biomedical Informatics Group, a nonprofit group, represents the interests of a broad range of clinical and non-clinical professionals working within the Health Informatics sphere. Its purposes are:

- Promote the implementation of the computer tool in the healthcare activity, scientific research, health administration and in all areas related to health sciences and biomedical research.

- Support, promote and disseminate content related activities with the management of health information and tools they used to do under the name of Biomedical informatics.

- Promote cooperation and exchange of actions generated in the field of biomedical informatics, both in the public and private, national and international level.

- Interact with all scientists, recognized academic stimulating the creation of new instances that have the same goal and be inspired by the same purpose.

- To promote, organize, sponsor and participate in events and activities for training in computer and information and disseminating developments in this area that might be useful for team members and health related activities.

The Argentinian health system is heterogeneous in its function, and because of that the informatics developments show a heterogeneous stage. Many private Health Care center have developed systems, such as the Hospital Aleman of Buenos Aires, or the Hospital Italiano de Buenos Aires that also has a residence program for health informatics.

Brazil

The first applications of computers to medicine and healthcare in Brazil started around 1968, with the installation of the first mainframes in public university hospitals, and the use of programmable calculators in scientific research applications. Minicomputers, such as the IBM 1130 were installed in several universities, and the first applications were developed for them, such as the hospital census in the School of Medicine of Ribeirão Preto and patient master files, in the Hospital das Clínicas da Universidade de São Paulo, respectively at the cities of Ribeirão Preto and São Paulo campuses of the University of São Paulo. In the 1970s, several Digital Corporation and Hewlett Packard minicomputers were acquired for public and Armed Forces hospitals, and more intensively used for intensive-care unit, cardiology diagnostics, patient monitoring and other applications. In the early 1980s, with the arrival of cheaper microcomputers, a great upsurge of computer applications in health ensued, and in 1986 the Brazilian Society of Health Informatics was founded, the first Brazilian Congress of Health Informatics was held, and the first *Brazilian Journal of Health Informatics* was published. In Brazil, two universities are pioneers in teaching and research in Medical Informatics, both the University of Sao Paulo and the Federal University of Sao Paulo offer undergraduate programs highly qualified in the area as well as extensive graduate programs (MSc and PhD). In 2015 the Universidade Federal de Ciências da Saúde de Porto Alegre, Rio Grande do Sul, also started to offer undergraduate program.

Canada

Health Informatics projects in Canada are implemented provincially, with different provinces creating different systems. A national, federally funded, not-for-profit organization called Canada Health Infoway was created in 2001 to foster the development and adoption of electronic health records across Canada. As of December 31, 2008 there were 276 EHR projects under way in Canadian hospitals, other health-care facilities, pharmacies and laboratories, with an investment value of $1.5-billion from Canada Health Infoway.

Provincial and territorial programmes include the following:

- eHealth Ontario was created as an Ontario provincial government agency in September 2008. It has been plagued by delays and its CEO was fired over a multimillion-dollar contracts scandal in 2009.

- Alberta Netcare was created in 2003 by the Government of Alberta. Today the netCARE portal is used daily by thousands of clinicians. It provides access to demographic data, prescribed/dispensed drugs, known allergies/intolerances, immunizations, laboratory test results, diagnostic imaging reports, the diabetes registry and other medical reports. netCARE interface capabilities are being included in electronic medical record products which are being funded by the provincial government.

United States

In 2004, President George W. Bush signed Executive Order 13335, creating the Office of the National Coordinator for Health Information Technology (ONCHIT) as a division of the U.S. Department of Health and Human Services (HHS). The mission of this office is widespread adoption of interoperable electronic health records (EHRs) in the US within 10 years.

In 2014 The Department of Education approved an advanced Health Informatics Undergraduate program that was submitted by The University of South Alabama. The program is designed to provide specific Health Informatics education, and is the only program in the country with a Health

Informatics Lab. The program is housed in The School of Computing in Shelby Hall, a recently completed $50 million state of the art teaching facility. The University of South Alabama awarded David L. Loeser on May 10, 2014 with the first Health Informatics degree. The program currently is scheduled to have 100+ students awarded by 2016.

The Certification Commission for Healthcare Information Technology (CCHIT), a private non-profit group, was funded in 2005 by the U.S. Department of Health and Human Services to develop a set of standards for electronic health records (EHR) and supporting networks, and certify vendors who meet them. In July 2006, CCHIT released its first list of 22 certified ambulatory EHR products, in two different announcements.

Harvard Medical School added a department of biomedical informatics in 2015. The University of Cincinnati in partnership with Cincinnati Children's Medical Center created a biomedical informatics (BMI) Graduate certificate program and in 2015 began a BMI PhD program. The joint program allows for researchers and students to observe the impact their work has on patient care directly as discoveries are translated from bench to bedside.

Europe

The European Union's Member States are committed to sharing their best practices and experiences to create a European eHealth Area, thereby improving access to and quality health care at the same time as stimulating growth in a promising new industrial sector. The European eHealth Action Plan plays a fundamental role in the European Union's strategy. Work on this initiative involves a collaborative approach among several parts of the Commission services. The European Institute for Health Records is involved in the promotion of high quality electronic health record systems in the European Union.

UK

There are different models of health informatics delivery in each of the home countries (England, Scotland, Northern Ireland and Wales) but some bodies like UKCHIP operate for those 'in and for' all the home countries and beyond.

England

NHS informatics in England was contracted out to several vendors for national health informatics solutions under the National Programme for Information Technology (NPfIT) label in the early to mid-2000's, under the auspices of NHS Connecting for Health (part of the Health and Social Care Information Centre as of 1 April 2013). NPfIT originally divided the country into five regions, with strategic 'systems integration' contracts awarded to one of several Local Service Providers (LSP). The various specific technical solutions were required to connect securely with the NHS 'Spine', a system designed to broker data between different systems and care settings. NPfIT fell significantly behind schedule and its scope and design were being revised in real time, exacerbated by media and political lambasting of the Programme's spend (past and projected) against proposed budget. In 2010 a consultation was launched as part of the new Conservative/Liberal Democrat Coalition Government's White Paper 'Liberating the NHS'. This initiative provided little in the way of innovative thinking, primarily re-stating existing strategies within the proposed new context of the Coalition's vision for the NHS. The degree of computerisation in NHS secondary care was quite high before NPfIT, and the programme stagnated further development of the install base - the original NPfIT regional approach provided neither a single, nationwide solution nor local health community agility or autonomy to purchase systems, but instead tried to deal with a hinterland in the middle. Almost all general practices in England and Wales are computerised under the 'GP Systems of Choice' (GPSoC) programme, and patients have relatively extensive computerised primary care clinical records. System choice is the responsibility of individual general practices and while there is no single, standardised GP system, GPSoC sets relatively rigid minimum standards of performance and functionality for vendors to adhere to. Interoperation between primary and secondary care systems is rather primitive. It is hoped that a focus on interworking (for interfacing and integration) standards will stimulate synergy between primary and secondary care in sharing necessary information to support the care of individuals. Notable successes to date are in the electronic requesting and viewing of test results, and in some areas GPs have access to digital X-ray images from secondary care systems. Scotland has an approach to central connection under way which is more advanced than the English one in some ways. Scotland has the GPASS system whose source code is owned by the State, and controlled and developed by NHS Scotland. GPASS was accepted in 1984. It has been provided free to all GPs in Scotland but has developed poorly. Discussion of open sourcing it as a remedy is occurring.

Wales

Wales has a dedicated Health Informatics function that supports NHS Wales in leading on the new integrated digital information services and promoting Health Informatics as a career.

Netherlands

In the Netherlands, health informatics is currently a priority for research and implementation. The Netherlands Federation of University medical centers (NFU) has created the *Citrienfonds*, which includes the programs eHealth and Registration at the Source. The Netherlands also has the national organizations Society for Healthcare Informatics (VMBI) and Nictiz, the national center for standardization and eHealth.

Emerging Directions (European R&D)

The European Commission's preference, as exemplified in the 5th Framework as well as currently pursued pilot projects, is for Free/Libre and Open Source Software (FLOSS) for healthcare. Another stream of research currently focuses on aspects of "big data" in health information systems.

Asia and Oceania

In Asia and Australia-New Zealand, the regional group called the Asia Pacific Association for Medical Informatics (APAMI) was established in 1994 and now consists of more than 15 member regions in the Asia Pacific Region.

Australia

The Australasian College of Health Informatics (ACHI) is the professional association for health informatics in the Asia-Pacific region. It represents the interests of a broad range of clinical and non-clinical professionals working within the health informatics sphere through a commitment to quality, standards and ethical practice. ACHI is an academic institutional member of the International Medical Informatics Association (IMIA) and a full member of the Australian Council of Professions. ACHI is a sponsor of the "e-Journal for Health Informatics", an indexed and peer-reviewed professional journal. ACHI has also supported the "Australian Health Informatics Education Council" (AHIEC) since its founding in 2009.

Although there are a number of health informatics organisations in Australia, the Health Informatics Society of Australia (HISA) is regarded as the major umbrella group and is a member of the International Medical Informatics Association (IMIA). Nursing informaticians were the driving force behind the formation of HISA, which is now a company limited by guarantee of the members. The membership comes from across the informatics spectrum that is from students to corporate affiliates. HISA has a number of branches (Queensland, New South Wales, Victoria and Western Australia) as well as special interest groups such as nursing (NIA), pathology, aged and community care, industry and medical imaging (Conrick, 2006).

China

After 20 years, China performed a successful transition from its planned economy to a socialist market economy. Along this change, China's healthcare system also experienced a significant reform to follow and adapt to this historical revolution. In 2003, the data (released from Ministry of Health of the People's Republic of China (MoH)), indicated that the national healthcare-involved expenditure was up to RMB 662.33 billion totally, which accounted for about 5.56% of nationwide gross domestic products. Before the 1980s, the entire healthcare costs were covered in central government annual budget. Since that, the construct of healthcare-expended supporters started to change gradually. Most of the expenditure was contributed by health insurance schemes and private spending, which corresponded to 40% and 45% of total expenditure, respectively. Meanwhile, the financially governmental contribution was decreased to 10% only. On the other hand, by 2004, up to 296,492 healthcare facilities were recorded in statistic summary of MoH, and an average of 2.4 clinical beds per 1000 people were mentioned as well.

In China

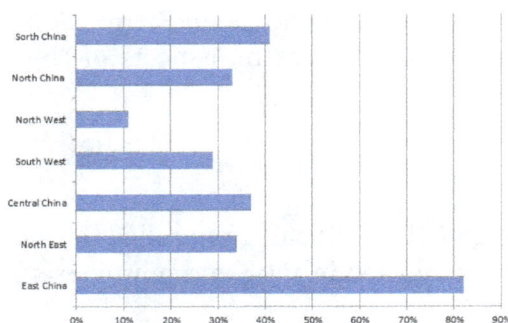

Proportion of Nationwide Hospitals with HIS in China by 2004

Along with the development of information technology since the 1990s, healthcare providers re-alised that the information could generate significant benefits to improve their services by com-puterised cases and data, for instance of gaining the information for directing patient care and as-sessing the best patient care for specific clinical conditions. Therefore, substantial resources were collected to build China's own health informatics system. Most of these resources were arranged to construct hospital information system (HIS), which was aimed to minimise unnecessary waste and repetition, subsequently to promote the efficiency and quality-control of healthcare. By 2004, China had successfully spread HIS through approximately 35–40% of nationwide hospitals. How-ever, the dispersion of hospital-owned HIS varies critically. In the east part of China, over 80% of hospitals constructed HIS, in northwest of China the equivalent was no more than 20%. Moreover, all of the Centers for Disease Control and Prevention (CDC) above rural level, approximately 80% of healthcare organisations above the rural level and 27% of hospitals over town level have the ability to perform the transmission of reports about real-time epidemic situation through public health information system and to analysis infectious diseases by dynamic statistics.

China has four tiers in its healthcare system. The first tier is street health and workplace clinics and these are cheaper than hospitals in terms of medical billing and act as prevention centers. The second tier is district and enterprise hospitals along with specialist clinics and these provide the second level of care. The third tier is provisional and municipal general hospitals and teaching hospitals which provided the third level of care. In a tier of its own is the national hospitals which are governed by the Ministry of Health. China has been greatly improving its health informatics since it finally opened its doors to the outside world and joined the World Trade Organization (WTO). In 2001, it was reported that China had 324,380 medical institutions and the majority of those were clinics. The reason for that is that clinics are prevention centers and Chinese people like using traditional Chinese medicine as opposed to Western medicine and it usually works for the minor cases. China has also been im-proving its higher education in regards to health informatics. At the end of 2002, there were 77 med-ical universities and medical colleges. There were 48 university medical colleges which offered bach-elor, master, and doctorate degrees in medicine. There were 21 higher medical specialty institutions that offered diploma degrees so in total, there were 147 higher medical and educational institutions. Since joining the WTO, China has been working hard to improve its education system and bring it up to international standards. SARS played a large role in China quickly improving its healthcare system. Back in 2003, there was an outbreak of SARS and that made China hurry to spread HIS or Hospital Information System and more than 80% of hospitals had HIS. China had been comparing itself to Korea's healthcare system and figuring out how it can better its own system. There was a study done that surveyed six hospitals in China that had HIS. The results were that doctors didn't use computers as much so it was concluded that it wasn't used as much for clinical practice than it was for administrative purposes. The survey asked if the hospitals created any websites and it was concluded that only four of them had created websites and that three had a third-party company cre-ate it for them and one was created by the hospital staff. In conclusion, all of them agreed or strongly agreed that providing health information on the Internet should be utilized.

Standards in China

Collected information at different times, by different participants or systems could frequently lead to issues of misunderstanding, dis-comparing or dis-exchanging. To design an issues-minor sys-tem, healthcare providers realised that certain standards were the basis for sharing information and interoperability, however a system lacking standards would be a large impediment to interfere the improvement of corresponding information systems. Given that the standardisation for health informatics depends on the authorities, standardisation events must be involved with government and the subsequently relevant funding and supports were critical. In 2003, the Ministry of Health released the Development Lay-out of National Health Informatics (2003–2010) indicating the identification of standardisation for health informatics which is 'combining adoption of international standards and development of national standards'.

In China, the establishment of standardisation was initially facilitated with the development of vocabulary, classification and coding, which is conducive to reserve and transmit information for premium management at national level. By 2006, 55 international/ domestic standards of vocabulary, classification and coding have served in hospital information system. In 2003, the 10th revision of the International Statistical Classification of Diseases and Related Health Problems (ICD-10) and the ICD-10 Clinical Modification (ICD-10-CM) were adopted as standards for diagnostic classification and acute care procedure classification. Simultaneously, the International Classification of Primary Care (ICPC) were translated and tested in China 's local applied environment. Another coding standard, named Logical Observation Identifiers Names and Codes (LOINC), was applied to serve as general identifiers for clinical observation in hospitals. Personal identifier codes were widely employed in different information systems, involving name, sex, nationality, family relationship, educational level and job occupation. However, these codes within different systems are inconsistent, when sharing between different regions. Considering this large quantity of vocabulary, classification and coding standards between different jurisdictions, the healthcare provider realised that using multiple systems could generate issues of resource wasting and a non-conflicting national level standard was beneficial and necessary. Therefore, in late 2003, the health informatics group in Ministry of Health released three projects to deal with issues of lacking national health information standards, which were the Chinese National Health Information Framework and Standardisation, the Basic Data Set Standards of Hospital Information System and the Basic Data Set Standards of Public Health Information System.

Objectives of Chinese National Health Information Framework and Standardisation

1. Establish national health information framework and identify in what areas standards and guidelines are required

2. Identify the classes, relationships and attributes of national health information framework. Produce a conceptual health data model to cover the scope of the health information framework

3. Create logical data model for specific domains, depicting the logical data entities, the data attributes, and the relationships between the entities according to the conceptual health data model

4. Establish uniform represent standard for data elements according to the data entities and their attributes in conceptual data model and logical data model

5. Circulate the completed health information framework and health data model to the partnership members for review and acceptance

6. Develop a process to maintain and refine the China model and to align with and influence international health data models

Comparison between China's EHR Standard and Segments of the ASTM E 1384 Standard

Recently, researchers from local universities evaluated the performance of China's Electronic Health Record(EHR) Standard compared with the American Society for Testing and Materials Standard Practice for Content and Structure of Electronic Health Records in the United States (ASTM E 1384 Standard).

China'sEHR standard	ASTM E 1384 standard
• H.01 Document identifier, H.02 Service object identifier, H.03 Demographics, H.04 Contact person, H.05 Address, H.06 Contacts	• Seg1 Demographic/Administrative, Seg14A Administrative/Diagnostic
• H.07 Medical insurance	
• H.08 Healthcare institution, H.09 Healthcare practitioner	• Seg4 Provider/Practitioners
• H.10 Event summary	• Seg5 Problem List, Seg14A Administrative/Diagnostic Summary
• S.01 Chief complaints	• Seg14B Chief Complaint Present Illness/Trauma Care
• S.02 Physical exam	• Seg9 Assessments/Exams
• S.03 Present illness history	• Seg14B Chief Complaint Present Illness/Trauma Care
• S.04 Past medical history	• Seg5 Problem List, Seg6 Immunizations, Seg7 Exposure to Hazardous Substances, Seg8 Family/Prenatal/Cumulative Health/Medical/Dental Nursing History
• S.05 Specific Exam, S.06 Lab data	• Seg11 Diagnostic Tests
• S.07 Diagnoses	• Seg5 Problem List, Seg14A Administrative/Diagnostic Summary
• S.08 Procedures	• Seg14E Procedures
• S.09 Medications	• Seg12 Medications
• S.10 Care/treatment plans	• Seg2 Legal Agreements, Seg10 Care/Treatment Plans and Orders, Seg13 Scheduled Appointments/Events
• S.11 Assessments	• Seg9 Assessments/Exams
• S.12 Encounters/episodes notes	• Seg14C Progress Notes/Clinical Course, Seg14D Therapies, Seg14F Disposition
• S.13 Financial information	• Seg3 Financial
• S.14 Nursing service	• Seg8 Family/Prenatal/Cumulative Health/Medical/Dental Nursing History, Seg14D Therapies
• S.15 Health guidance	• Seg10 Care/Treatment Plans and Orders
• S.16 Four diagnostic methods in Traditional Chinese medicine	• Seg11 Diagnostic Tests

The table above demonstrates details of this comparison which indicates certain domains of improvement for future revisions of EHR Standard in China. Detailedly, these deficiencies are listed in the following.

1. The lack of supporting on privacy and security. The ISO/TS 18308 specifies "The EHR must support the ethical and legal use of personal information, in accordance with established privacy principles and frameworks, which may be culturally or jurisdictionally

specific" (ISO 18308: Health Informatics-Requirements for an Electronic Health Record Architecture, 2004). However this China's EHR Standard did not achieve any of the fifteen requirements in the subclass of privacy and security.

2. The shortage of supporting on different types of data and reference. Considering only ICD-9 is referenced as China's external international coding systems, other similar systems, such as SNOMED CT in clinical terminology presentation, cannot be considered as familiar for Chinese specialists, which could lead to internationally information-sharing deficiency.

3. The lack of more generic and extensible lower level data structures. China's large and complex EHR Standard was constructed for all medical domains. However, the specific and time-frequent attributes of clinical data elements, value sets and templates identified that this once-for-all purpose cannot lead to practical consequence.

Hong Kong

In Hong Kong a computerized patient record system called the Clinical Management System (CMS) has been developed by the Hospital Authority since 1994. This system has been deployed at all the sites of the authority (40 hospitals and 120 clinics). It is used for up to 2 million transactions daily by 30,000 clinical staff. The comprehensive records of 7 million patients are available on-line in the electronic patient record (ePR), with data integrated from all sites. Since 2004 radiology image viewing has been added to the ePR, with radiography images from any HA site being available as part of the ePR.

The Hong Kong Hospital Authority placed particular attention to the governance of clinical systems development, with input from hundreds of clinicians being incorporated through a structured process. The health informatics section in the Hospital Authority has a close relationship with the information technology department and clinicians to develop healthcare systems for the organization to support the service to all public hospitals and clinics in the region.

The Hong Kong Society of Medical Informatics (HKSMI) was established in 1987 to promote the use of information technology in healthcare. The eHealth Consortium has been formed to bring together clinicians from both the private and public sectors, medical informatics professionals and the IT industry to further promote IT in healthcare in Hong Kong.

Malaysia

Since 2010, the Ministry of Health (MoH) has been working on the Malaysian Health Data Warehouse (MyHDW) project. MyHDW aims to meet the diverse needs of timely health information provision and management, and acts as a platform for the standardization and integration of health data from a variety of sources (Health Informatics Centre, 2013). The Ministry has embarked on introducing the electronic Hospital Information Systems (HIS) in several public hospitals including Serdang Hospital, Selayang Hospital and University Kebangsaan Malaysia Medical Centre (UKMMC) under the Ministry of Higher Education (MOHE).

A hospital information system (HIS) is a comprehensive, integrated information system designed to manage the administrative, financial and clinical aspects of a hospital. As an area of medical informatics, the aim of hospital information system is to achieve the best possible support of patient care and administration by electronic data processing. HIS plays a vital role in planning, initiating, organizing and controlling the operations of the subsystems of the hospital and thus provides a synergistic organization in the process.

New Zealand

Health informatics is taught at five New Zealand universities. The most mature and established programme has been offered for over a decade at Otago. Health Informatics New Zealand (HINZ), is the national organisation that advocates for health informatics. HINZ organises a conference every year and also publishes a journal- *Healthcare Informatics Review Online.*

Saudi Arabia

The Saudi Association for Health Information (SAHI) was established in 2006 to work under direct supervision of King Saud bin Abdulaziz University for Health Sciences to practice public activities, develop theoretical and applicable knowledge, and provide scientific and applicable studies.

Post Soviet Countries

The Russian Federation

The Russian healthcare system is based on the principles of the Soviet healthcare system, which was oriented on mass prophylaxis, prevention of infection and epidemic diseases, vaccination and immunization of the population on a socially protected basis. The current government healthcare system consists of several directions:

- Preventive health care
- Primary health care
- Specialized medical care
- Obstetrical and gynecologic medical care
- Pediatric medical care
- Surgery
- Rehabilitation/ Health resort treatment

One of the main issues of the post-Soviet medical health care system was the absence of the united system providing optimization of work for medical institutes with one, single database and structured appointment schedule and hence hours-long lines. Efficiency of medical workers might have been also doubtful because of the paperwork administrating or lost book records.

Along with the development of the information systems IT and healthcare departments in Moscow agreed on design of a system that would improve public services of health care institutes. Tackling the issues appearing in the existing system, the Moscow Government ordered that the design of a system would provide simplified electronic booking to public clinics and automate the work of medical workers on the first level.

The system designed for that purposes was called EMIAS (United Medical Information and Analysis System) and presents an electronic health record (EHR) with the majority of other services set in the system that manages the flow of patients, contains outpatient card integrated in the system, and provides an opportunity to manage consolidated managerial accounting and personalized list of medical help. Besides that, the system contains information about availability of the medical institutions and various doctors.

The implementation of the system started in 2013 with the organization of one computerized database for all patients in the city, including a front-end for the users. EMIAS was implemented in Moscow and the region and it is planned that the project should extend to most parts of the country.

Law

Health informatics law deals with evolving and sometimes complex legal principles as they apply to information technology in health-related fields. It addresses the privacy, ethical and operational issues that invariably arise when electronic tools, information and media are used in health care delivery. Health Informatics Law also applies to all matters that involve information technology, health care and the interaction of information. It deals with the circumstances under which data and records are shared with other fields or areas that support and enhance patient care.

As many healthcare systems are making an effort to have patient records more readily available to them via the internet, it is important that providers implement security standards in order to ensure that the patients' information is safe. They have to be able to assure confidentiality, integrity, and security of the people, process, and technology. Since there is also the possibility of payments being made through this system, it is vital that this aspect of their private information will also be protected through cryptography.

The use of technology in health care settings has become popular and this trend is expected to continue. Various healthcare facilities had instigated different kinds of health information technology systems in the provision of patient care, such as electronic health records (EHRs), computerized charting, etc. The growing popularity of health information technology systems and the escalation in the amount of health information that can be exchanged and transferred electronically increased the risk of potential infringement in patients' privacy and confidentiality. This concern triggered the establishment of strict measures by both policymakers and individual facility to ensure patient privacy and confidentiality.

One of the federal laws enacted to safeguard patient's health information (medical record, billing information, treatment plan, etc.) and to guarantee patient's privacy is the Health Insurance Portability and Accountability Act of 1996 or HIPAA. HIPAA gives patients the autonomy and control over their own health records. Furthermore, according to the U.S. Department of Health & Human Services (n.d.), this law enables patients to do the following:

- Allows patients to view their own health records

- Permits patients to request for a copy of their own medical records

- Modify any incorrect health information

- Provides patients with the right to know as to who have access to their health record

- Grants patients the right to request who can and cannot view/access their health information

Leading Health Informatics and Medical Informatics Journals

Computers in Biomedical and Research, published in 1967 was one of the first dedicated journals to health informatics. Some additional early journals included Computers and Medicine published by the American Medical Association, Journal of Clinical Computing, published by Gallagher Printing, Journal of Medical Systems, published by Plenum Press, and MD computing, published by Springer-Veriag. In 1984, Lippincott published the first nursing specific journal titled, Journal Computers in Nursing which is now known as Computers Informatics Nursing (CIN) Journal. Today, there are many health and medical informatics journals. As of September 7, 2016, there are roughly 235 informatics journals listed in the National Library of Medicine (NLM) catalog of journals. Here is a list of some of the top health and medical informatics journals:

- Journal of Medical Internet Research

- JMIR mHealth and uHealth

- JMIR Medical Informatics

- JMIR Human Factors

- JMIR Public Health & Surveillance

- Journal of the American Medical Informatics Association : JAMIA

- International Journal of Medical Informatics

- Implementation Science

- Medical Image Analysis

- Medical Decision Making

- Journal of Biomedical Informatics

- BMC Medical Research Methodology

- Artificial Intelligence in Medicine

- CIN: Computers Informatics Nursing

Health Policy

Health policy can be defined as the "decisions, plans, and actions that are undertaken to achieve specific healthcare goals within a society. According to the World Health Organization, an explicit health policy can achieve several things: it defines a vision for the future; it outlines priorities and the expected roles of different groups; and it builds consensus and informs people.

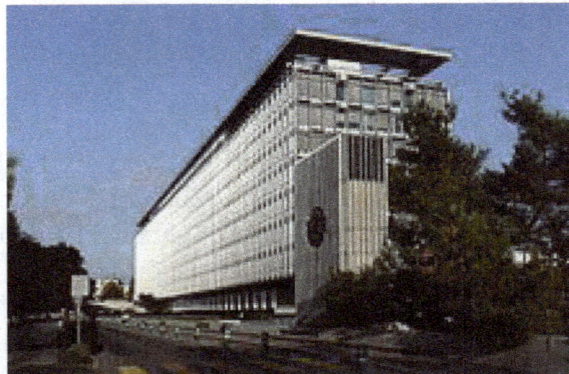

The headquarters of the World Health Organization in Geneva, Switzerland.

There are many categories of health policies, including global health policy, public health policy, mental health policy, health care services policy, insurance policy, personal healthcare policy, pharmaceutical policy, and policies related to public health such as vaccination policy, tobacco control policy or breastfeeding promotion policy. They may cover topics of financing and delivery of healthcare, access to care, quality of care, and health equity.

Background

Health-related policy and its implementation is complex. Conceptual models can help show the flow from health-related policy development to health-related policy and program implementation and to health systems and health outcomes. Policy should be understood as more than a national law or health policy that supports a program or intervention. Operational policies are the rules, regulations, guidelines, and administrative norms that governments use to translate national laws and policies into programs and services. The policy process encompasses decisions made at a national or decentralized level (including funding decisions) that affect whether and how services are delivered. Thus, attention must be paid to policies at multiple levels of the health system and over time to ensure sustainable scale-up. A supportive policy environment will facilitate the scale-up of health interventions.

There are many topics in the politics and evidence that can influence the decision of a government, private sector business or other group to adopt a specific policy. Evidence-based policy relies on the use of science and rigorous studies such as randomized controlled trials to identify programs and practices capable of improving policy relevant outcomes. Most political debates surround personal health care policies, especially those that seek to reform healthcare delivery, and can typically be categorized as either philosophical or economic. Philosophical debates center around questions about individual rights, ethics and government authority, while economic topics include how to maximize the efficiency of health care delivery and minimize costs.

The modern concept of healthcare involves access to medical professionals from various fields as well as medical technology, such as medications and surgical equipment. It also involves access to the latest information and evidence from research, including medical research and health services research.

In many countries it is left to the individual to gain access to healthcare goods and services by paying for them directly as out-of-pocket expenses, and to private sector players in the medical and pharmaceutical industries to develop research. Planning and production of health human resources is distributed among labour market participants.

Other countries have an explicit policy to ensure and support access for all of its citizens, to fund health research, and to plan for adequate numbers, distribution and quality of health workers to meet healthcare goals. Many governments around the world have established universal health care, which takes the burden of healthcare expenses off of private businesses or individuals through pooling of financial risk. There are a variety of arguments for and against universal healthcare and related health policies. Healthcare is an important part of health systems and therefore it often accounts for one of the largest areas of spending for both governments and individuals all over the world.

Personal Healthcare Policy Options

Philosophy: Right to Health

Many countries and jurisdictions integrate a human rights philosophy in directing their healthcare policies. The World Health Organization reports that every country in the world is party to at least one human rights treaty that addresses health-related rights, including the right to health as well as other rights that relate to conditions necessary for good health. The United Nations' Universal Declaration of Human Rights (UDHR) asserts that medical care is a right of all people:

- *UDHR Article 25:* "Everyone has the right to a standard of living adequate for the health and well-being of himself and of his family, including food, clothing, housing and medical care and necessary social services, and the right to security in the event of unemployment, illness, disability, widowhood, old age or other lack of livelihood in circumstances beyond his control."

In some jurisdictions and among different faith-based organizations, health policies are influenced by the perceived obligation shaped by religious beliefs to care for those in less favorable circumstances, including the sick. Other jurisdictions and non-governmental organizations draw on the principles of humanism in defining their health policies, asserting the same perceived obligation and enshrined right to health. In recent years, the worldwide human rights organization Amnesty International has focused on health as a human right, addressing inadequate access to HIV drugs and women's sexual and reproductive rights including wide disparities in maternal mortality within and across countries. Such increasing attention to health as a basic human right has been welcomed by the leading medical journal *The Lancet*.

There remains considerable controversy regarding policies on who would be paying the costs of medical care for all people and under what circumstances. For example, government spending on healthcare is sometimes used as a global indicator of a government's commitment to the health of its people. On the other hand, one school of thought emerging from the United States rejects the notion of health care financing through taxpayer funding as incompatible with the (considered no less important) right of the physician's professional judgment, and the related concerns that government involvement in overseeing the health of its citizens could erode the right to privacy between doctors and patients. The argument furthers that universal health insurance denies the right of individual patients to dispose of their own income as per their own will.

Another issue in the rights debate is governments' use of legislation to control competition among private medical insurance providers against national social insurance systems, such as the case in Canada's national health insurance program. Laissez-faire supporters argue that this erodes the cost-effectiveness of the health system, as even those who can afford to pay for private healthcare services drain resources from the public system. The issue here is whether investor-owned medical insurance companies or health maintenance organizations are in a better position to act in the best interests of their customers compared to government regulation and oversight. Another claim in the United States perceives government over-regulation of the healthcare and insurance industries as the effective end of charitable home visits from doctors among the poor and elderly.

Economics: Healthcare Financing

Many types of health policies exist focusing on the financing of healthcare services to spread the economic risks of ill health. These include publicly funded health care (through taxation or insurance, also known as single-payer systems), mandatory or voluntary private health insurance, and complete capitalization of personal health care services through private companies, among others. The debate is ongoing on which type of health financing policy results in better or worse quality of healthcare services provided, and how to ensure allocated funds are used effectively, efficiently and equitably.

There are many arguments on both sides of the issue of public versus private health financing policies:

Claims that publicly funded healthcare improves the quality and efficiency of personal health care delivery:

- Government spending on health is essential for the accessibility and sustainability of healthcare services and programmes.

- For those people who would otherwise go without care due to lack of financial means, any quality care is an improvement.

- Since people perceive universal healthcare as *free* (if there is no insurance premium or co-payment), they are more likely to seek preventive care which may reduce the disease burden and overall healthcare costs in the long run.

- Single-payer systems reduce wastefulness by removing the middle man, i.e. private insurance companies, thus reducing the amount of bureaucracy. In particular, reducing the amount of paperwork that medical professionals have to deal with for insurance claims processing allows them to concentrate more on treating patients.

Claims that privately funded healthcare leads to greater quality and efficiencies in personal health care:

- Perceptions that publicly funded healthcare is *free* can lead to overuse of medical services, and hence raise overall costs compared to private health financing.

- Privately funded medicine leads to greater quality and efficiencies through increased access to and reduced waiting times for specialized health care services and technologies.

- Limiting the allocation of public funds for personal healthcare does not curtail the ability of uninsured citizens to pay for their healthcare as out-of-pocket expenses. Public funds can be better rationalized to provide emergency care services regardless of insured status or ability to pay, such as with the Emergency Medical Treatment and Active Labor Act in the United States.

- Privately funded and operated healthcare reduces the requirement for governments to increase taxes to cover healthcare costs, which may be compounded by the inefficiencies among government agencies due to their greater bureaucracy.

Other Health Policy Options

Health policy options extend beyond the financing and delivery of personal health care, to domains such as medical research and health workforce planning, both domestically and internationally.

Medical Research Policy

Medical research can be both the basis for defining evidence-based health policy, and the subject of health policy itself, particularly in terms of its sources of funding. Those in favor of government policies for publicly funded medical research posit that removing profit as a motive will increase the rate of medical innovation. Those opposed argue that it will do the opposite, because removing the incentive of profit removes incentives to innovate and inhibits new technologies from being developed and utilized.

The existence of sound medical research does not necessarily lead to evidence-based policymaking. For example, in South Africa, whose population sets the record for HIV infections, previous government policy limiting funding and access for AIDS treatments met with strong controversy given its basis on a refusal to accept scientific evidence on the means of transmission. A change of government eventually led to a change in policy, with new policies implemented for widespread access to HIV services. Another issue relates to intellectual property, as illustrated by the case of Brazil, where debates have arisen over government policy authorizing the domestic manufacture of antiretroviral drugs used in the treatment of HIV/AIDS in violation of drug patents.

Health Workforce Policy

Some countries and jurisdictions have an explicit policy or strategy to plan for adequate numbers, distribution and quality of health workers to meet healthcare goals, such as to address physician and nursing shortages. Elsewhere, workforce planning is distributed among labour market participants as a laissez-faire approach to health policy. Evidence-based policies for workforce development are typically based on findings from health services research.

Health in Foreign Policy

Many governments and agencies include a health dimension in their foreign policy in order to achieve global health goals. Promoting health in lower income countries has been seen as instrumental to achieve other goals on the global agenda, including:

- Promoting global security – linked to fears of global pandemics, the intentional spread of pathogens, and a potential increase in humanitarian conflicts, natural disasters, and emergencies;

- Promoting economic development – including addressing the economic effect of poor health on development, of pandemic outbreaks on the global market place, and also the gain from the growing global market in health goods and services;

- Promoting social justice – reinforcing health as a social value and human right, including supporting the United Nations' Millennium Development Goals.

Global Health Policy

Global health policy encompasses the global governance structures that create the policies underlying public health throughout the world. In addressing global health, global health policy "implies consideration of the health needs of the people of the whole planet above the concerns of particular nations." Distinguished from both international health policy (agreements among sovereign states) and comparative health policy (analysis of health policy across states), global health policy institutions consist of the actors and norms that frame the global health response.

Disease Management (Health)

Disease management is defined as "a system of coordinated healthcare interventions and communications for populations with conditions in which patient self-care efforts are significant."

For people who can access health care practitioners or peer support it is the process whereby persons with long-term conditions (and often family/friend/carer) share knowledge, responsibility and care plans with healthcare practitioners and/or peers. To be effective it requires whole system implementation with community social support networks, a range of satisfying occupations and activities relevant to the context, clinical professionals willing to act as partners or coaches and on-line resources which are verified and relevant to the country and context. Knowledge sharing, knowledge building and a learning community are integral to the concept of disease management. It is a population health strategy as well as an approach to personal health. It may reduce healthcare costs and/or improve quality of life for individuals by preventing or minimizing the effects of disease, usually a chronic condition, through knowledge, skills, enabling a sense of control over life (despite symptoms of disease) and integrative care.

History

Disease management has evolved from managed care, specialty capitation, and health service demand management, and refers to the processes and people concerned with improving or maintaining health in large populations. It is concerned with common chronic illnesses, and the reduction of future complications associated with those diseases.

Illnesses that disease management would concern itself with would include: coronary heart disease, chronic obstructive pulmonary disease (COPD), kidney failure, hypertension, heart failure, obesity, diabetes mellitus, asthma, cancer, arthritis, clinical depression, sleep apnea, osteoporosis, and other common ailments.

Industry

In the United States, disease management is a large industry with many vendors. Major disease management organizations based on revenues and other criteria include Accordant (a subsidiary of Caremark), Alere (now including ParadigmHealth and Matria Healthcare), Caremark (excluding its Accordant subsidiary), Evercare, Health Dialog, Healthways, LifeMasters (now part of StayWell), LifeSynch (formerly Corphealth), Magellan, McKesson Health Solutions, and MedAssurant.

Disease management is of particular importance to health plans, agencies, trusts, associations and employers that offer health insurance. A 2002 survey found that 99.5% of enrollees of Health Maintenance Organization/Point Of Service (HMO/POS) plans are in plans that cover at least one disease management program. A Mercer Consulting study indicated that the percentage of employer-sponsored health plans offering disease management programs grew to 58% in 2003, up from 41% in 2002.

It was reported that $85 million was spent on disease management in the United States in 1997, and $600 million in 2002. Between 2000 and 2005, the compound annual growth rate of revenues for disease management organizations was 28%. In 2000, the Boston Consulting Group estimated that the U.S. market for outsourced disease management could be $20 billion by 2010; however, in 2008 the Disease Management Purchasing Consortium estimated that disease management organization revenues would be $2.8 billion by 2010. As of 2010, a study using National Ambulatory Medical Care Survey data estimated that 21.3% of patients in the U.S. with at least one chronic condition use disease management programs. Yet, management of chronic conditions is responsible for more than 75% of all health care spending.

Process

The underlying premise of disease management is that when the right tools, ...experts, and equipment are applied to a population, labor costs (specifically: absenteeism, presenteeism, and direct insurance expenses) can be minimized in the near term, or resources can be provided more efficiently. The general idea is to ease the disease path, rather than cure the disease. Improving quality and activities for daily living are first and foremost. Improving cost, in some programs, is a necessary component, as well. However, some disease management systems believe that reductions in longer term problems may not be measureable today, but may warrant continuation of disease management programs until better data is available in 10–20 years. Most disease management vendors offer return on investment (ROI) for their programs, although over the years there have been dozens of ways to measure ROI. Responding to this inconsistency, an industry trade association, the Care Continuum Alliance, convened industry leaders to develop consensus guidelines for measuring clinical and financial outcomes in disease management, wellness and other population-based programs. Contributing to the work were public and private health and quality organizations, including the federal Agency for Healthcare Research and Quality, the National Committee for Quality Assurance, URAC, and the Joint Commission. The project produced the first volume of a now four-volume Outcomes Guidelines Report, which details industry-consensus approaches to measuring outcomes.

Tools include web-based assessment tools, clinical guidelines, health risk assessments, outbound and inbound call-center-based triage, best practices, formularies, and numerous other devices, systems and protocols.

Experts include actuaries, physicians, pharmacists, medical economists, nurses, nutritionists, physical therapists, statisticians, epidemiologists, and human resources professionals. Equipment can include mailing systems, web-based applications (with or without interactive modes), monitoring devices, or telephonic systems.

Effectiveness

Possible Biases

When disease management programs are voluntary, studies of their effectiveness may be affected by a self-selection bias; that is, a program may "attract enrollees who were [already] highly motivated to succeed". At least two studies have found that people who enroll in disease management programs differ significantly from those who do not on baseline clinical, demographic, cost, utilization and quality parameters. To minimize any bias in estimates of the effectiveness of disease management due to differences in baseline characteristics, randomized controlled trials are better than observational studies.

Even if a particular study is a randomized trial, it may not provide strong evidence for the effectiveness of disease management. A 2009 review paper examined randomized trials and meta-analyses of disease management programs for heart failure and asserted that many failed the PICO process and Consolidated Standards of Reporting Trials: "interventions and comparisons are not sufficiently well described; that complex programs have been excessively oversimplified; and that potentially salient differences in programs, populations, and settings are not incorporated into analyses."

Medicare

Section 721 of the Medicare Prescription Drug, Improvement, and Modernization Act of 2003 authorized the Centers for Medicare and Medicaid Services (CMS) to conduct what became the "Medicare Health Support" project to examine disease management. Phase I of the project involved disease management companies (such as Aetna Health Management, CIGNA Health Support, Health Dialog Services Corp., Healthways, and McKesson Health Solutions) chosen by a competitive process in eight states and the District of Columbia. The project focused on people with diabetes or heart failure who had relatively high Medicare payments; in each location, approximately 20,000 such people were randomly assigned to an intervention group and 10,000 were randomly assigned to a control group. CMS set goals in the areas of clinical quality and beneficiary satisfaction, and negotiated with the disease management programs for a target of 5% savings in Medicare costs. The programs started between August 2005 and January 2006. What is now the Care Continuum Alliance praised the project as "the first-ever national pilot integrating sophisticated care management techniques into the Medicare fee-for-service program".

An initial evaluation of Phase I of the project by RTI International appeared in June 2007 which had "three key participation and financial findings":

- Medicare expenditures for the intervention group were higher than those of the comparison group by the time the pilots started.

- Within the intervention group, participants had lower Medicare payments (i.e., tended to be healthier) than non-participants.

- The "fees paid to date far exceed any savings produced."

DMAA focused on another finding of the initial evaluation, the "high levels of satisfaction with chronic disease management services among beneficiaries and physicians". One commentary noted that the project "can only be observational" since "equivalence was not achieved at baseline". Another commentary claimed that the project was "in big trouble". A paper on the six-month evaluation, published in fall 2008, concluded that "Results to date indicate limited success in achieving Medicare cost savings or reducing acute care utilization".

In December 2007, CMS changed the financial threshold from 5% savings to budget neutrality, a change that DMAA "hailed". In January 2008, however, CMS decided to end Phase I because it claimed that the statutory authority had run out. Four U.S. senators wrote a letter to CMS to reverse its decision. DMAA decried the termination of Phase I and called upon CMS to start Phase II as soon as possible. Among other criticisms of the project, the disease management companies claimed that Medicare "signed up patients who were much sicker than they had expected," failed to transmit information on patients' prescriptions and laboratory results to them in a timely fashion, and disallowed the companies from selecting patients most likely to benefit from disease management.

By April 2008, CMS had spent $360 million on the project. The individual programs ended between December 2006 and August 2008.

The results of the program were published in *The New England Journal of Medicine* in November 2011. Comparing the 163,107 patients randomized to the intervention group with the 79,310 patients randomized to the control group, the researchers found that "disease-management programs did not reduce hospital admissions or emergency room visits, as compared with usual care." Furthermore, there was "no demonstrable savings in Medicare expenditures," with the net fees for disease management ranging from 3.8% to 10.9% per patient per month. The researchers suggested that the findings might be explained by the severity of chronic disease among the patients studied, delays in patients' receiving disease management after hospitalizations, and lack of integration between health coaches and the patients' primary care providers.

Other Studies

Studies that have reviewed other studies on the effectiveness of disease management include the following:

- A 2004 Congressional Budget Office analysis concluded that published studies "do not provide a firm basis for concluding that disease management programs generally reduce total costs". The report caused the disease management industry to "scrambl[e] to build a better business case for their services".

- A 2005 review of 44 studies on disease management found a positive return on investment (ROI) for congestive heart failure and multiple disease conditions, but inconclusive, mixed, or negative ROI for diabetes, asthma, and depression management programs. The lead author, of Cornell University and Thomson Medstat, was quoted as saying that the paucity of research conducted on the ROI of disease management was "a concern because so many companies and government agencies have adopted disease management to manage the cost of care for people with chronic conditions."

- A 2007 RAND summary of 26 reviews and meta-analyses of small-scale disease management programs, and 3 evaluations of population-based disease management programs, concluded that "Payers and policy makers should remain skeptical about vendor claims [concerning disease management] and should demand supporting evidence based on transparent and scientifically sound methods." In specific:

  o Disease management improved "clinical processes of care" (e.g., adherence to evidence-based guidelines) for congestive heart failure, coronary artery disease, diabetes, and depression.

  o There was inconclusive evidence, insufficient evidence, or evidence for no effect of disease management on health-related behaviors.

  o Disease management led to better disease control for congestive heart failure, coronary artery disease, diabetes, and depression.

  o There was inconclusive evidence, insufficient evidence, or evidence for no effect of disease management on clinical outcomes (e.g., "mortality and functional status").

  o Disease management reduced hospital admission rates for congestive heart failure, but increased health care utilization for depression, with inconclusive or insufficient evidence for the other diseases studied.

  o In the area of financial outcomes, there was inconclusive evidence, insufficient evidence, evidence for no effect, or evidence for increased costs.

  o Disease management increased patient satisfaction and health-related quality of life in congestive heart failure and depression, but the evidence was insufficient for the other diseases studied.

  A subsequent letter to the editor claimed that disease management might nevertheless "satisfy buyers today, even if academics remain unconvinced".

- A 2008 systematic review and meta-analysis concluded that disease management for COPD "modestly improved exercise capacity, health-related quality of life, and hospital admissions, but not all-cause mortality".

- A 2009 review of 27 studies "could not draw definitive conclusions about the effectiveness or cost-effectiveness of... asthma disease-management programs" for adults.

- A Canadian systematic review published in 2009 found that home telehealth in chronic disease management may be cost-saving but that "the quality of the studies was generally low."

- Researchers from The Netherlands systematically reviewed 31 papers published 2007–2009 and determined that the evidence that disease management programs for four diseases reduce healthcare expenditures is "inconclusive."

- A meta-analysis of randomized trials published through 2009 estimated that disease management for diabetes has "a clinically moderate but significant impact on hemoglobin A_{1C} levels," with an absolute mean difference of 0.51% between experimental and control groups.

- A 2011 "meta-review" (systematic review of meta-analyses) of heart failure disease management programs found them to be of "mixed quality" in that they did not report important characteristics of the studies reviewed.

Recent studies not reviewed in the aforementioned papers include the following:

- A U.K. study published in 2007 found certain improvements in the care of patients with coronary artery disease and heart failure (e.g., better management of blood pressure and cholesterol) if they received nurse-led disease management instead of usual care.

- In a 2007 Canadian study, people were randomized to receive or not receive disease management for heart failure for a period of six months. Emergency room visits, hospital readmissions, and all-cause deaths were no different in the two groups after 2.8 years of follow-up.

- A 2008 U.S. study found that nurse-led disease management for patients with heart failure was "reasonably cost-effective" per quality-adjusted life year compared with a "usual care group".

- A 2008 study from the Netherlands compared no disease management with "basic" nurse-led disease management with "intensive" nurse-led disease management for patients discharged from the hospital with heart failure; it detected no significant differences in hospitalization and death for the three groups of patients.

- A retrospective cohort study from 2008 found that disease management did not increase the use of drugs recommended for patients after a heart attack.

- Of 15 care coordination (disease management) programs followed for two years in a 2008 study, "few programs improved patient behaviors, health, or quality of care" and "no program reduced gross or net expenditures".

- After 18 months, a 2008 Florida study found "virtually no overall impacts on hospital or emergency room (ER) use, Medicare expenditures, quality of care, or prescription drug use" for a disease management program.

- With minor exceptions, a paper published in 2008 did not find significant differences in outcomes among people with asthma randomly assigned to telephonic disease management, augmented disease management (including in-home respiratory therapist visits), or traditional care.

- A 2009 review by the Centers for Medicare and Medicaid Services of 35 disease management programs that were part of demonstration projects between 1999 and 2008 found that relatively few improved quality in a budget-neutral manner.

- In a 2009 randomized trial, high- and moderate-intensity disease management did not improve smoking cessation rates after 24 months compared with drug therapy alone.

- A randomized trial published in 2010 determined that disease management reduced a composite score of emergency room visits and hospitalizations among patients discharged from Veterans Administration hospitals for chronic obstructive pulmonary disease. A 2011 post-hoc analysis of the study's data estimated that the intervention produced a net cost savings of $593 per patient.

- A Spanish study published in 2011 randomized 52 people hospitalized for heart failure to follow-up with usual care, 52 to home visits, 52 to telephone follow-up, and 52 to an in-hospital heart failure unit. After a median of 10.8 months of follow-up, there were no significant differences in hospitalization or mortality among the four groups.

- Among 18- to 64-year-old people with chronic diseases receiving Medicaid, telephone-based disease management in one group of members did not reduce ambulatory care visits, hospitalizations, or expenditures relative to a control group. Furthermore, in this 2011 study, the group receiving disease management had a lower decrease in emergency department visits than the group not receiving disease management.

Public Health

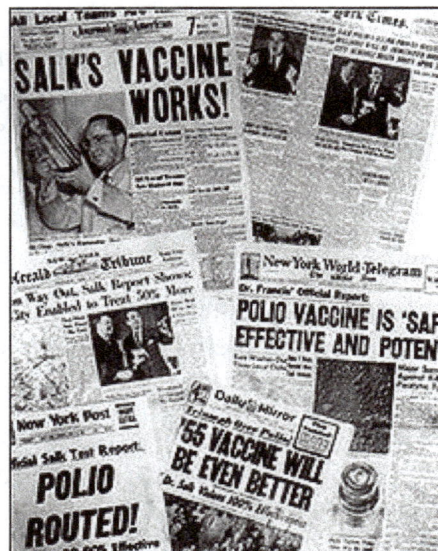

Newspaper headlines from around the world about polio vaccine tests (13 April 1955)

Public health refers to "the science and art of preventing disease, prolonging life and promoting human health through organized efforts and informed choices of society, organizations, public and private, communities and individuals." It is concerned with threats to health based on population health analysis. The population in question can be as small as a handful of people, or as large as all the inhabitants of several continents (for instance, in the case of a pandemic). The dimensions of health can encompass "a state of complete physical, mental and social well-being and not merely the absence of disease or infirmity," as defined by the United Nations' World Health Organization. Public health incorporates the interdisciplinary approaches of epidemiology, biostatistics and health services. Environmental health, community health, behavioral health, health economics, public policy, mental health and occupational safety and health are other important subfields.

The focus of public health intervention is to improve health and quality of life through prevention and treatment of disease and other physical and mental health conditions. This is done through surveillance of cases and health indicators, and through promotion of healthy behaviors. Examples of common public health measures include promotion of hand washing, breastfeeding, delivery of vaccinations, suicide prevention and distribution of condoms to control the spread of sexually transmitted diseases.

Modern public health practice requires multidisciplinary teams of public health workers and professionals including the following: physicians specializing in public health, community medicine, or infectious disease; psychologists; epidemiologists; biostatisticians; medical assistants or Assistant Medical Officers; public health nurses; midwives; medical microbiologists; environmental health officers or public health inspectors; pharmacists; dentists; dietitians and nutritionists; veterinarians; public health engineers; public health lawyers; sociologists; community development workers; communications experts; bioethicists; and others.

There is a great disparity in access to health care and public health initiatives between developed nations and developing nations. In the developing world, public health infrastructures are still forming.

Background

The focus of a public health intervention is to prevent and manage diseases, injuries and other health conditions through surveillance of cases and the promotion of healthy behaviors, communities and environments. Many diseases are preventable through simple, nonmedical methods. For example, research has shown that the simple act of hand washing with soap can prevent many contagious diseases. In other cases, treating a disease or controlling a pathogen can be vital to preventing its spread to others, either during an outbreak of infectious disease or through contamination of food or water supplies. Public health communications programs, vaccination programs and distribution of condoms are examples of common public health measures. Measures such as these have contributed greatly to the health of populations and increases in life expectancy.

Public health plays an important role in disease prevention efforts in both the developing world and in developed countries, through local health systems and non-governmental organizations. The World Health Organization (WHO) is the international agency that coordinates and acts on global public health issues. Most countries have their own government public health agencies, sometimes known as ministries of health, to respond to domestic health issues. For example, in the United States, the front line of public health initiatives are state and local health departments. The United States Public Health Service (PHS), led by the Surgeon General of the United States, and the Centers for Disease Control and Prevention, headquartered in Atlanta, are involved with several international health activities, in addition to their national duties. In Canada, the Public Health Agency of Canada is the national agency responsible for public health, emergency preparedness and response, and infectious and chronic disease control and prevention. The Public health system in India is managed by the Ministry of Health & Family Welfare of the government of India with state-owned health care facilities.

Current practice

Public Health Programs

There's a push and pull, as you know, between cheap alternatives for industry and public health concerns...We're always looking at retrospectively what the data shows...Unfortunately, for example, take tobacco: It took 50, 60 years of research before policy catches up with what the science is showing— Laura Anderko, professor at Georgetown University and director of the Mid-Atlantic Center for Children's Health and the Environment commenting on public health practices in response to proposal to ban chlorpyrifos pesticide.

Most governments recognize the importance of public health programs in reducing the incidence of disease, disability, and the effects of aging and other physical and mental health conditions, although public health generally receives significantly less government funding compared with medicine. Public health programs providing vaccinations have made strides in promoting health, including the eradication of smallpox, a disease that plagued humanity for thousands of years.

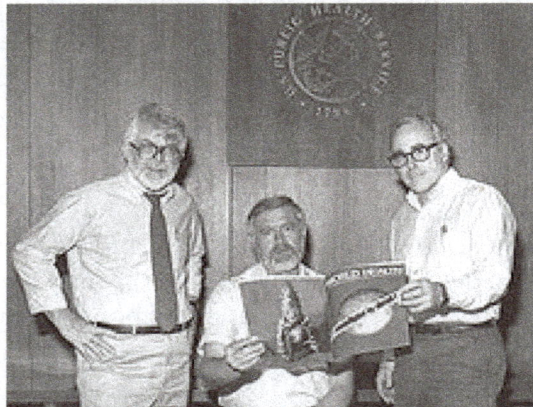

Three former directors of the Global Smallpox Eradication Programme read the news
that smallpox had been globally eradicated, 1980

The World Health Organization (WHO) identifies core functions of public health programs including:

- providing leadership on matters critical to health and engaging in partnerships where joint action is needed;

- shaping a research agenda and stimulating the generation, translation and dissemination of valuable knowledge;

- setting norms and standards and promoting and monitoring their implementation;

- articulating ethical and evidence-based policy options;

- monitoring the health situation and assessing health trends.

In particular, public health surveillance programs can:

- serve as an early warning system for impending public health emergencies;

- document the impact of an intervention, or track progress towards specified goals; and

- monitor and clarify the epidemiology of health problems, allow priorities to be set, and inform health policy and strategies.

- diagnose, investigate, and monitor health problems and health hazards of the community

Public health surveillance has led to the identification and prioritization of many public health issues facing the world today, including HIV/AIDS, diabetes, waterborne diseases, zoonotic diseases, and antibiotic resistance leading to the reemergence of infectious diseases such as tuberculosis. Antibiotic resistance, also known as drug resistance, was the theme of World Health Day 2011. Although the prioritization of pressing public health issues is important, Laurie Garrett argues that there are following consequences. When foreign aid is funnelled into disease-specific programs, the importance of public health in general is disregarded. This public health problem of stovepiping is thought to create a lack of funds to combat other existing diseases in a given country.

For example, the WHO reports that at least 220 million people worldwide suffer from diabetes. Its incidence is increasing rapidly, and it is projected that the number of diabetes deaths will double by the year 2030. In a June 2010 editorial in the medical journal *The Lancet*, the authors opined that "The fact that type 2 diabetes, a largely preventable disorder, has reached epidemic proportion is a public health humiliation." The risk of type 2 diabetes is closely linked with the growing problem of obesity. The WHO's latest estimates highlighted that globally approximately 1.5 billion adults were overweight in 2008, and nearly 43 million children under the age of five were overweight in 2010. The United States is the leading country with 30.6% of its population being obese. Mexico follows behind with 24.2% and the United Kingdom with 23%. Once considered a problem in high-income countries, it is now on the rise in low-income countries, especially in urban settings. Many public health programs are increasingly dedicating attention and resources to the issue of obesity, with objectives to address the underlying causes including healthy diet and physical exercise.

Some programs and policies associated with public health promotion and prevention can be controversial. One such example is programs focusing on the prevention of HIV transmission through safe sex campaigns and needle-exchange programmes. Another is the control of tobacco smoking. Changing smoking behavior requires long-term strategies, unlike the fight against communicable diseases, which usually takes a shorter period for effects to be observed. Many nations have implemented major initiatives to cut smoking, such as increased taxation and bans on smoking in some or all public places. Proponents argue by presenting evidence that smoking is one of the major killers, and that therefore governments have a duty to reduce the death rate, both through limiting passive (second-hand) smoking and by providing fewer opportunities for people to smoke. Opponents say that this undermines individual freedom and personal responsibility, and worry that the state may be emboldened to remove more and more choice in the name of better population health overall.

Simultaneously, while communicable diseases have historically ranged uppermost as a global health priority, non-communicable diseases and the underlying behavior-related risk factors have been at the bottom. This is changing however, as illustrated by the United Nations hosting its first General Assembly Special Summit on the issue of non-communicable diseases in September 2011.

Many health problems are due to maladaptive personal behaviors. From an evolutionary psychology perspective, over consumption of novel substances that are harmful is due to the activation of an evolved reward system for substances such as drugs, tobacco, alcohol, refined salt, fat, and carbohydrates. New technologies such as modern transportation also cause reduced physical activity. Research has found that behavior is more effectively changed by taking evolutionary motivations into consideration instead of only presenting information about health effects. Thus, the increased use of soap and hand-washing to prevent diarrhea is much more effectively promoted if its lack of use is associated with the emotion of disgust. Disgust is an evolved system for avoiding contact with substances that spread infectious diseases. Examples might include films that show how fecal matter contaminates food. The marketing industry has long known the importance of associating products with high status and attractiveness to others. Conversely, it has been argued that emphasizing the harmful and undesirable effects of tobacco smoking on other persons and imposing smoking bans in public places have been particularly effective in reducing tobacco smoking.

Applications in Health Care

As well as seeking to improve population health through the implementation of specific population-level interventions, public health contributes to medical care by identifying and assessing population needs for health care services, including:

- Assessing current services and evaluating whether they are meeting the objectives of the health care system

- Ascertaining requirements as expressed by health professionals, the public and other stakeholders

- Identifying the most appropriate interventions

- Considering the effect on resources for proposed interventions and assessing their cost-effectiveness

- Supporting decision making in health care and planning health services including any necessary changes.

- Informing, educating, and empowering people about health issues

Implementing Effective Improvement Strategies

To improve public health, one important strategy is to promote modern medicine and scientific neutrality to drive the public health policy and campaign, which is recommended by Armanda Solorzana, through a case study of the Rockefeller Foundation's hookworm campaign in Mexico in the 1920s. Soloranza argues that public health policy can't concern only politics or economics. Political concerns can lead government officials to hide the real numbers of people affected by disease in their regions, such as upcoming elections. Therefore, scientific neutrality in making public health policy is critical; it can ensure treatment needs are met regardless of political and economic conditions.

The history of public health care clearly shows the global effort to improve health care for all. However, in modern-day medicine, real, measurable change has not been clearly seen, and critics argue that this lack of improvement is due to ineffective methods that are being implemented. As argued by Paul E. Farmer, structural interventions could possibly have a large impact, and yet there are numerous problems as to why this strategy has yet to be incorporated into the health system. One of the main reasons that he suggests could be the fact that physicians are not properly trained to carry out structural interventions, meaning that the ground level health care professionals cannot implement these improvements. While structural interventions can not be the only area for improvement, the lack of coordination between socioeconomic factors and health care for the poor could be counterproductive, and end up causing greater inequity between the health care services received by the rich and by the poor. Unless health care is no longer treated as a commodity, global public health can ultimately not be achieved. This being the case, without changing the way in which health care is delivered to those who have less access to it, the universal goal of public health care cannot be achieved.

Public Health 2.0

Public Health 2.0 is a movement within public health that aims to make the field more accessible to the general public and more user-driven. The term is used in three senses. In the first sense, "Public Health 2.0" is similar to "Health 2.0" and describes the ways in which traditional public health practitioners and institutions are reaching out (or could reach out) to the public through social media and health blogs.

In the second sense, "Public Health 2.0" describes public health research that uses data gathered from social networking sites, search engine queries, cell phones, or other technologies. A recent example is the proposal of statistical framework that utilizes online user-generated content (from social media or search engine queries) to estimate the impact of an influenza vaccination campaign in the UK.

In the third sense, "Public Health 2.0" is used to describe public health activities that are completely user-driven. An example is the collection and sharing of information about environmental radiation levels after the March 2011 tsunami in Japan. In all cases, Public Health 2.0 draws on ideas from Web 2.0, such as crowdsourcing, information sharing, and user-centred design. While many individual healthcare providers have started making their own personal contributions to "Public Health 2.0" through personal blogs, social profiles, and websites, other larger organizations, such as the American Heart Association (AHA) and United Medical Education (UME), have a larger team of employees centered around online driven health education, research, and training. These private organizations recognize the need for free and easy to access health materials often building libraries of educational articles.

Developing Countries

There is a great disparity in access to health care and public health initiatives between developed nations and developing nations. In the developing world, public health infrastructures are still forming. There may not be enough trained health workers or monetary resources to provide even a basic level of medical care and disease prevention. As a result, a large majority of disease and mortality in the developing world results from and contributes to extreme poverty. For example, many African governments spend less than US$10 per person per year on health care, while, in the United States, the federal government spent approximately US$4,500 per capita in 2000. However, expenditures on health care should not be confused with spending on public health. Public health measures may not generally be considered "health care" in the strictest sense. For example, mandating the use of seat belts in cars can save countless lives and contribute to the health of a population, but typically money spent enforcing this rule would not count as money spent on health care.

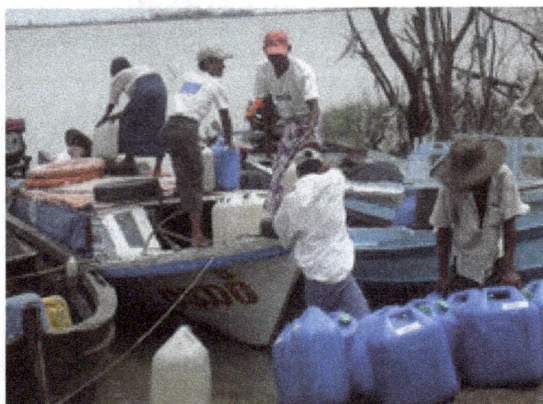

Emergency Response Team in Burma after Cyclone Nargis in 2008

Large parts of the developing world remained plagued by largely preventable or treatable infectious diseases and poor maternal and child health, exacerbated by malnutrition and poverty. The WHO reports that a lack of exclusive breastfeeding during the first six months of life contributes to over a million avoidable child deaths each year. Intermittent preventive therapy aimed at treating and preventing malaria episodes among pregnant women and young children is one public health measure in endemic countries.

Each day brings new front-page headlines about public health: emerging infectious diseases such as SARS, rapidly making its way from China to Canada, the United States and other geographically distant countries; reducing inequities in health care access through publicly funded health insurance programs; the HIV/AIDS pandemic and its spread from certain high-risk groups to the general population in many countries, such as in South Africa; the increase of childhood obesity and the concomitant increase in type II diabetes among children; the social, economic and health effects of adolescent pregnancy; and the public health challenges related to natural disasters such as the 2004 Indian Ocean tsunami, 2005's Hurricane Katrina in the United States and the 2010 Haiti earthquake.

Since the 1980s, the growing field of population health has broadened the focus of public health from individual behaviors and risk factors to population-level issues such as inequality, poverty, and education. Modern public health is often concerned with addressing determinants of health across a population. There is a recognition that our health is affected by many factors including where we live, genetics, our income, our educational status and our social relationships; these are known as "social determinants of health." A social gradient in health runs through society. The poorest generally suffer the worst health, but even the middle classes will generally have worse health outcomes than those of a higher social stratum. The new public health advocates for population-based policies that improve health in an equitable manner.

Sustainable Development Goals

To address current and future challenges in addressing health issues in the world, the United Nations have developed the Sustainable Development Goals 2015 building off of the Millennium Development Goals of 2000 to be completed by 2030. These goals in their entirety encompass the entire spectrum of development across nations, however Goals 1-6 directly address health disparities, primarily in developing countries. These six goals address key issues in global public health: Poverty, Hunger and food security, Health, Education, Gender equality and women's empowerment, and water and sanitation. Public health officials can use these goals to set their own agenda and plan for smaller scale initiatives for their organizations. These goals hope to lessen the burden of disease and inequality faced by developing countries and lead to a healthier future.

The links between the various sustainable development goals and public health are numerous and well established:

- Living below the poverty line is attributed to poorer health outcomes and can be even worse for persons living in developing countries where extreme poverty is more common. A child born into poverty is twice as likely to die before the age of five compared to a child from a wealthier family.

- The detrimental effects of hunger and malnutrition that can arise from systemic challenges with food security are enormous. The World Health Organization estimates that 12.9 percent of the population in developing countries is undernourished.

- Health challenges in the developing world are enormous, with "only half of the women in developing nations receiving the recommended amount of healthcare they need.

- Educational equity has yet to be reached in the world. Public health efforts are impeded by this, as a lack of education can lead to poorer health outcomes. This is shown by children of mothers who have no education having a lower survival rate compared to children born to mothers with primary or greater levels of education. Cultural differences in the role of women vary by country, many gender inequalities are found in developing nations. Combating these inequalities has shown to also lead to better public health outcome.

- In studies done by the World Bank on populations in developing countries, it was found that when women had more control over household resources, the children benefit through better access to food, healthcare, and education.

- Basic sanitation resources and access to clean sources of water are a basic human right. However, 1.8 billion people globally use a source of drinking water that is fecally contaminated, and 2.4 billion people lack access to basic sanitation facilities like toilets or pit latrines. A lack of these resources is what causes approximately 1000 children a day to die from diarrhoel diseases that could have been prevented from better water and sanitation infrastructure.

Education and Training

Education and training of public health professionals is available throughout the world in Schools of Public Health, Medical Schools, Veterinary Schools, Schools of Nursing, and Schools of Public

Affairs. The training typically requires a university degree with a focus on core disciplines of bio-statistics, epidemiology, health services administration, health policy, health education, behavioral science and environmental health. In the global context, the field of public health education has evolved enormously in recent decades, supported by institutions such as the World Health Organization and the World Bank, among others. Operational structures are formulated by strategic principles, with educational and career pathways guided by competency frameworks, all requiring modulation according to local, national and global realities. It is critically important for the health of populations that nations assess their public health human resource needs and develop their ability to deliver this capacity, and not depend on other countries to supply it.

Schools of Public Health - a U.S. Perspective

In the United States, the Welch-Rose Report of 1915 has been viewed as the basis for the critical movement in the history of the institutional schism between public health and medicine because it led to the establishment of schools of public health supported by the Rockefeller Foundation. The report was authored by William Welch, founding dean of the Johns Hopkins Bloomberg School of Public Health, and Wickliffe Rose of the Rockefeller Foundation. The report focused more on research than practical education. Some have blamed the Rockefeller Foundation's 1916 decision to support the establishment of schools of public health for creating the schism between public health and medicine and legitimizing the rift between medicine's laboratory investigation of the mechanisms of disease and public health's nonclinical concern with environmental and social influences on health and wellness.

Even though schools of public health had already been established in Canada, Europe and North Africa, the United States had still maintained the traditional system of housing faculties of public health within their medical institutions. A $25,000 donation from businessman Samuel Zemurray instituted the School of Public Health and Tropical Medicine at Tulane University in 1912 conferring its first doctor of public health degree in 1914. The Johns Hopkins School of Hygiene and Public Health became an independent, degree-granting institution for research and training in public health, and the largest public health training facility in the United States, when it was founded in 1916. By 1922, schools of public health were established at Columbia, Harvard and Yale on the Hopkins model. By 1999 there were twenty nine schools of public health in the US, enrolling around fifteen thousand students.

Over the years, the types of students and training provided have also changed. In the beginning, students who enrolled in public health schools typically had already obtained a medical degree; public health school training was largely a second degree for medical professionals. However, in 1978, 69% of American students enrolled in public health schools had only a bachelor's degree.

Degrees in Public Health

Schools of public health offer a variety of degrees which generally fall into two categories: professional or academic. The two major postgraduate degrees are the Master of Public Health (M.P.H.) or the Master of Science in Public Health (MSPH). Doctoral studies in this field include Doctor of Public Health (DrPH) and Doctor of Philosophy (Ph.D.) in a subspeciality of greater Public Health disciplines. DrPH is regarded as a professional degree and Ph.D. as more of an academic degree.

Professional degrees are oriented towards practice in public health settings. The Master of Public Health, Doctor of Public Health, Doctor of Health Science (DHSc) and the Master of Health Care Administration are examples of degrees which are geared towards people who want careers as practitioners of public health in health departments, managed care and community-based organizations, hospitals and consulting firms among others. Master of Public Health degrees broadly fall into two categories, those that put more emphasis on an understanding of epidemiology and statistics as the scientific basis of public health practice and those that include a more eclectic range of methodologies. A Master of Science of Public Health is similar to an MPH but is considered an academic degree (as opposed to a professional degree) and places more emphasis on scientific methods and research. The same distinction can be made between the DrPH and the DHSc. The DrPH is considered a professional degree and the DHSc is an academic degree.

Academic degrees are more oriented towards those with interests in the scientific basis of public health and preventive medicine who wish to pursue careers in research, university teaching in graduate programs, policy analysis and development, and other high-level public health positions. Examples of academic degrees are the Master of Science, Doctor of Philosophy, Doctor of Science (ScD), and Doctor of Health Science (DHSc). The doctoral programs are distinct from the MPH and other professional programs by the addition of advanced coursework and the nature and scope of a dissertation research project.

In the United States, the Association of Schools of Public Health represents Council on Education for Public Health (CEPH) accredited schools of public health. Delta Omega is the honor society for graduate studies in public health. The society was founded in 1924 at the Johns Hopkins School of Hygiene and Public Health. Currently, there are approximately 68 chapters throughout the United States and Puerto Rico.

History

Early history

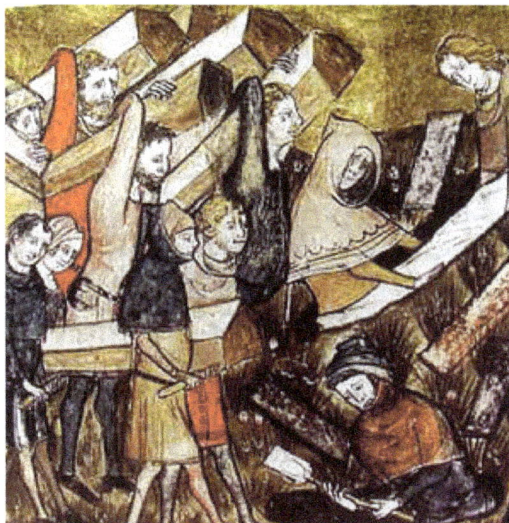

The primitive nature of medieval medicine rendered Europe helpless to the onslaught of the Black Death in the 14th century. Fragment of a miniature from "The Chronicles of Gilles Li Muisis" (1272-1352). Bibliothèque royale de Belgique, MS 13076-77, f. 24v.

Public health has early roots in antiquity. From the beginnings of human civilization, it was recognized that polluted water and lack of proper waste disposal spread communicable diseases (theory of miasma). Early religions attempted to regulate behavior that specifically related to health, from types of food eaten, to regulating certain indulgent behaviors, such as drinking alcohol or sexual relations. Leaders were responsible for the health of their subjects to ensure social stability, prosperity, and maintain order.

By Roman times, it was well understood that proper diversion of human waste was a necessary tenet of public health in urban areas. The ancient Chinese medical doctors developed the practice of variolation following a smallpox epidemic around 1000 BC. An individual without the disease could gain some measure of immunity against it by inhaling the dried crusts that formed around lesions of infected individuals. Also, children were protected by inoculating a scratch on their forearms with the pus from a lesion.

In 1485 the Republic of Venice established a Permanent Court of supervisors of health with special attention to the prevention of the spread of epidemics in the territory from abroad. The three supervisors were initially appointed by the Venetian Senate. In 1537 it was assumed by the Grand Council, and in 1556 added two judges, with the task of control, on behalf of the Republic, the efforts of the supervisors.

However, according to Michel Foucault, the plague model of governmentality was later controverted by the cholera model. A Cholera pandemic devastated Europe between 1829 and 1851, and was first fought by the use of what Foucault called "social medicine", which focused on flux, circulation of air, location of cemeteries, etc. All those concerns, born of the miasma theory of disease, were mixed with urbanistic concerns for the management of populations, which Foucault designated as the concept of "biopower". The German conceptualized this in the *Polizeiwissenschaft* ("Police science").

Modern Public Health

The 18th century saw rapid growth in voluntary hospitals in England. The latter part of the century brought the establishment of the basic pattern of improvements in public health over the next two centuries: a social evil was identified, private philanthropists brought attention to it, and changing public opinion led to government action.

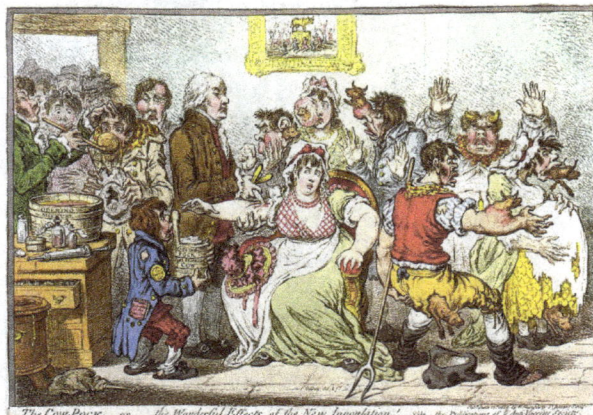

The Cow-Pock — or — the Wonderful Effects of the New Inoculation! — vid. the Publications of ye Anti-Vaccine Society

1802 caricature of Edward Jenner vaccinating patients who feared it would make them sprout cowlike appendages.

The practice of vaccination became prevalent in the 1800s, following the pioneering work of Edward Jenner in treating smallpox. James Lind's discovery of the causes of scurvy amongst sailors and its mitigation via the introduction of fruit on lengthy voyages was published in 1754 and led to the adoption of this idea by the Royal Navy. Efforts were also made to promulgate health matters to the broader public; in 1752 the British physician Sir John Pringle published *Observations on the Diseases of the Army in Camp and Garrison*, in which he advocated for the importance of adequate ventilation in the military barracks and the provision of latrines for the soldiers.

With the onset of the Industrial Revolution, living standards amongst the working population began to worsen, with cramped and unsanitary urban conditions. In the first four decades of the 19th century alone, London's population doubled and even greater growth rates were recorded in the new industrial towns, such as Leeds and Manchester. This rapid urbanisation exacerbated the spread of disease in the large conurbations that built up around the workhouses and factories. These settlements were cramped and primitive with no organized sanitation. Disease was inevitable and its incubation in these areas was encouraged by the poor lifestyle of the inhabitants. Unavailable housing led to the rapid growth of slums and the per capita death rate began to rise alarmingly, almost doubling in Birmingham and Liverpool. Thomas Malthus warned of the dangers of overpopulation in 1798. His ideas, as well as those of Jeremy Bentham, became very influential in government circles in the early years of the 19th century.

Public Health Legislation

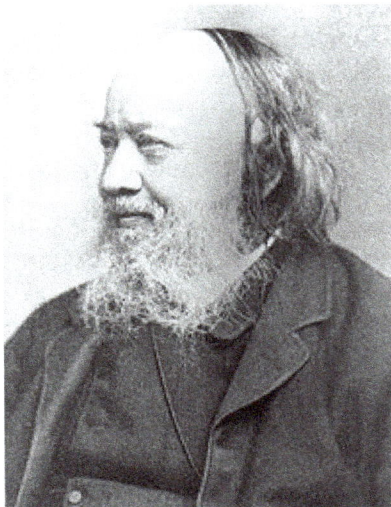

Sir Edwin Chadwick was a pivotal influence on the early public health campaign.

The first attempts at sanitary reform and the establishment of public health institutions were made in the 1840s. Thomas Southwood Smith, physician at the London Fever Hospital, began to write papers on the importance of public health, and was one of the first physicians brought in to give evidence before the Poor Law Commission in the 1830s, along with Neil Arnott and James Phillips Kay. Smith advised the government on the importance of quarantine and sanitary improvement for limiting the spread of infectious diseases such as cholera and yellow fever.

The Poor Law Commission reported in 1838 that "the expenditures necessary to the adoption and maintenance of measures of prevention would ultimately amount to less than the cost of the disease now constantly engendered". It recommended the implementation of large scale government engineering projects to alleviate the conditions that allowed for the propagation of disease. The Health of Towns Association was formed in Exeter on 11 December 1844, and vigorously campaigned for the development of public health in the United Kingdom. Its formation followed the 1843 establishment of the Health of Towns Commission, chaired by Sir Edwin Chadwick, which produced a series of reports on poor and insanitary conditions in British cities.

These national and local movements led to the Public Health Act, finally passed in 1848. It aimed to improve the sanitary condition of towns and populous places in England and Wales by placing the supply of water, sewerage, drainage, cleansing and paving under a single local body with the General Board of Health as a central authority. The Act was passed by the Liberal government of Lord John Russell, in response to the urging of Edwin Chadwick. Chadwick's seminal report on *The Sanitary Condition of the Labouring Population* was published in 1842 and was followed up with a supplementary report a year later.

Vaccination for various diseases was made compulsory in the United Kingdom in 1851, and by 1871 legislation required a comprehensive system of registration run by appointed vaccination officers.

Further interventions were made by a series of subsequent Public Health Acts, notably the 1875 Act. Reforms included latrinization, the building of sewers, the regular collection of garbage followed by incineration or disposal in a landfill, the provision of clean water and the draining of standing water to prevent the breeding of mosquitoes.

The Infectious Disease (Notification) Act 1889 mandated the reporting of infectious diseases to the local sanitary authority, which could then pursue measures such as the removal of the patient to hospital and the disinfection of homes and properties.

In the U.S., the first public health organization based on a state health department and local boards of health was founded in New York City in 1866.

Epidemiology

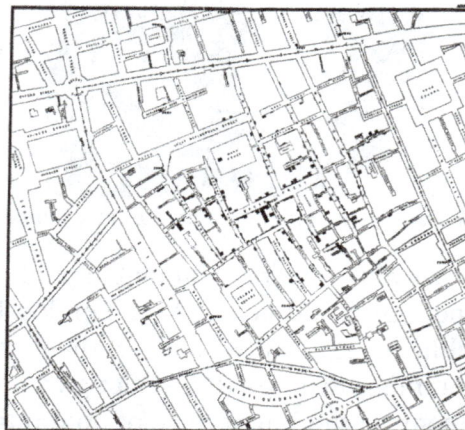

John Snow's dot map, showing the clusters of cholera cases in the London epidemic of 1854.

The science of epidemiology was founded by John Snow's identification of a polluted public water well as the source of an 1854 cholera outbreak in London. Dr. Snow believed in the germ theory of disease as opposed to the prevailing miasma theory. He first publicized his theory in an essay, *On the Mode of Communication of Cholera*, in 1849, followed by a more detailed treatise in 1855 incorporating the results of his investigation of the role of the water supply in the Soho epidemic of 1854.

By talking to local residents (with the help of Reverend Henry Whitehead), he identified the source of the outbreak as the public water pump on Broad Street (now Broadwick Street). Although Snow's chemical and microscope examination of a water sample from the Broad Street pump did not conclusively prove its danger, his studies of the pattern of the disease were convincing enough to persuade the local council to disable the well pump by removing its handle.

Snow later used a dot map to illustrate the cluster of cholera cases around the pump. He also used statistics to illustrate the connection between the quality of the water source and cholera cases. He showed that the Southwark and Vauxhall Waterworks Company was taking water from sewage-polluted sections of the Thames and delivering the water to homes, leading to an increased incidence of cholera. Snow's study was a major event in the history of public health and geography. It is regarded as the founding event of the science of epidemiology.

Disease Control

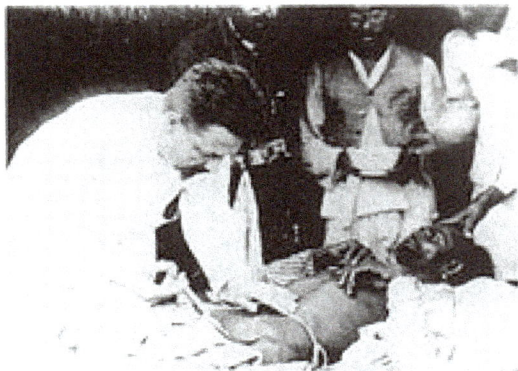

Paul-Louis Simond injecting a plague vaccine in Karachi, 1898.

With the pioneering work in bacteriology of French chemist Louis Pasteur and German scientist Robert Koch, methods for isolating the bacteria responsible for a given disease and vaccines for remedy were developed at the turn of the 20th century. British physician Ronald Ross identified the mosquito as the carrier of malaria and laid the foundations for combating the disease. Joseph Lister revolutionized surgery by the introduction of antiseptic surgery to eliminate infection. French epidemiologist Paul-Louis Simond proved that plague was carried by fleas on the back of rats, and Cuban scientist Carlos J. Finlay and U.S. Americans Walter Reed and James Carroll demonstrated that mosquitoes carry the virus responsible for yellow fever. Brazilian scientist Carlos Chagas identified a tropical disease and its vector.

With onset of the epidemiological transition and as the prevalence of infectious diseases decreased through the 20th century, public health began to put more focus on chronic diseases such as cancer and heart disease. Previous efforts in many developed countries had already led to dramatic reductions in the infant mortality rate using preventative methods. In Britain, the infant mortality rate fell from over 15% in 1870 to 7% by 1930.

Country Examples

France

France 1871-1914 followed well behind Bismarckian Germany, as well as Great Britain, in developing the welfare state including public health. Tuberculosis was the most dreaded disease of the day, especially striking young people in their 20s. Germany set up vigorous measures of public hygiene and public sanatoria, but France let private physicians handle the problem, which left it with a much higher death rate. The French medical profession jealously guarded its prerogatives, and public health activists were not as well organized or as influential as in Germany, Britain or the United States. For example, there was a long battle over a public health law which began in the 1880s as a campaign to reorganize the nation's health services, to require the registration of infectious diseases, to mandate quarantines, and to improve the deficient health and housing legislation of 1850. However the reformers met opposition from bureaucrats, politicians, and physicians. Because it was so threatening to so many interests, the proposal was debated and postponed for 20 years before becoming law in 1902. Success finally came when the government realized that contagious diseases had a national security impact in weakening military recruits, and keeping the population population growth rate well below Germany's.

United States

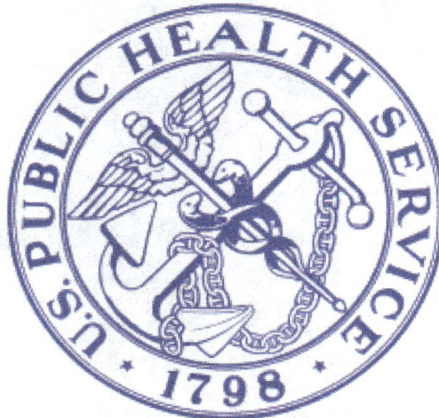

Seal of the United States Public Health Service

Most of the Public health activity in the United States took place at the municipal level before the mid-20th century. There was some activity at the national and state level as well.

In the administration of the second president of the United States John Adams, the Congress authorized the creation of hospitals for mariners. As the U.S. expanded, the scope of the governmental health agency expanded. In the United States, public health worker Sara Josephine Baker, M.D. established many programs to help the poor in New York City keep their infants healthy, leading teams of nurses into the crowded neighborhoods of Hell's Kitchen and teaching mothers how to dress, feed, and bathe their babies.

Another key pioneer of public health in the U.S. was Lillian Wald, who founded the Henry Street Settlement house in New York. The Visiting Nurse Service of New York was a significant organization for bringing health care to the urban poor.

Dramatic increases in average life span in the late 19th century and 20th century, is widely credited to public health achievements, such as vaccination programs and control of many infectious diseases including polio, diphtheria, yellow fever and smallpox; effective health and safety policies such as road traffic safety and occupational safety; improved family planning; tobacco control measures; and programs designed to decrease non-communicable diseases by acting on known risk factors such as a person's background, lifestyle and environment.

Another major public health improvement was the decline in the "urban penalty" brought about by improvements in sanitation. These improvements included chlorination of drinking water, filtration and sewage treatment which led to the decline in deaths caused by infectious waterborne diseases such as cholera and intestinal diseases. The federal Office of Indian Affairs (OIA) operated a large-scale field nursing program. Field nurses targeted native women for health education, emphasizing personal hygiene and infant care and nutrition.

Mexico

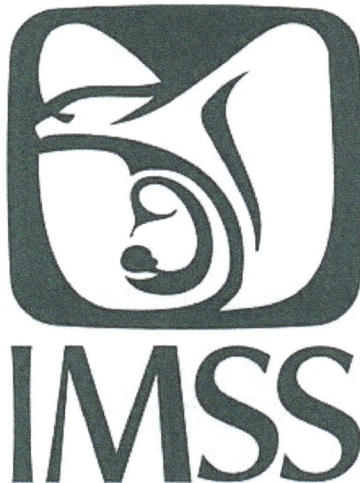

Logo for the Mexican Social Security Institute, a governmental agency dealing with public health.

Public health issues were important for the Spanish empire during the colonial era. Epidemic disease was the main factor in the decline of indigenous populations in the era immediately following the sixteenth-century conquest era and was a problem during the colonial era. The Spanish crown took steps in eighteenth-century Mexico to bring in regulations to make populations healthier.

In the late nineteenth century, Mexico was in the process of modernization, and public health issues were again tackled from a scientific point of view. Even during the Mexican Revolution (1910–20), public health was an important concern, with a text on hygiene published in 1916. During the Mexican Revolution, feminist and trained nurse Elena Arizmendi Mejia founded the Neutral White Cross, treating wounded soldiers no matter for what faction they fought.

In the post-revolutionary period after 1920, improved public health was a revolutionary goal of the Mexican government. The Mexican state promoted the health of the Mexican population, with most resources going to cities. Concern about disease conditions and social impediments to the improvement of Mexicans' health were important in the formation of the Mexican Society for Eugenics. The movement flourished from the 1920s to the 1940s. Mexico was not alone in Latin

America or the world in promoting eugenics. Government campaigns against disease and alcoholism were also seen as promoting public health.

The Mexican Social Security Institute was established in 1943, during the administration of President Manuel Avila Camacho to deal with public health, pensions, and social security.

Cuba

Since the 1959 Cuban Revolution the Cuban government has devoted extensive resources to the improvement of health conditions for its entire population via universal access to health care. Infant mortality has plummeted. Cuban medical internationalism as a policy has seen the Cuban government sent doctors as a form of aid and export to countries in need in Latin America, especially Venezuela, as well as Oceania and Africa countries.

Colombia and Bolivia

Public health was important elsewhere in Latin America in consolidating state power and integrating marginalized populations into the nation-state. In Colombia, public health was a means for creating and implementing ideas of citizenship. In Bolivia, a similar push came after their 1952 revolution.

Health Services Research

Health services research (HSR), also known as health systems research or health policy and systems research (HPSR), is a multidisciplinary scientific field that examines how people get access to health care practitioners and health care services, how much care costs, and what happens to patients as a result of this care. Studies in HSR investigate how social factors, health policy, financing systems, organizational structures and processes, medical technology, and personal behaviors affect access to health care, the quality and cost of health care, and quantity and quality of life. Compared with medical research, HSR is a relatively young science that developed through the bringing together of social science perspectives with the contributions of individuals and institutions engaged in delivering health services.

Goals

The primary goals of health services research are to identify the most effective ways to organize, manage, finance, and deliver high quality care; reduce medical errors; and improve patient safety. HSR is more concerned with delivery and access to care, in contrast to medical research, which focuses on the development and evaluation of clinical treatments.

Health services researchers come from a variety of specializations, including geography, nursing, economics, political science, epidemiology, public health, medicine, biostatistics, operations, management, engineering, pharmacy, psychology, usability and user experience design. While health services research is grounded in theory, its underlying aim is to perform research that can be applied by physicians, nurses, health managers and administrators, and other people who make decisions or deliver care in the health care system.

Approaches

Approaches to HSR include:

- *Implementation research*: research focusing on public policy analysis, or the concerns of program managers regarding the effectiveness of specific health interventions;

- *Impact evaluation*: research with emphasis on effectiveness of health care practices and organisation of care, using a more narrow range of study methods such as systematic reviews of health system interventions.

Health Services Research by country

Many data and information sources are used to conduct health services research, such as population and health surveys, clinical administrative records, health care program and financial administrative records, vital statistics records (births and deaths), and other special studies.

United States

Data Availability

Claims data on USA Medicare and Medicaid beneficiaries are available for analysis. Data is divided into public data available to any entity and research data available only to qualified researchers. USA's Centers for Medicare and Medicaid Services(CMS) delegates some data export functions to a Research Data Assistance Center.

23 Claims data from various states that are not limited to any particular insurer are also available for analysis via AHRQ's HCUP project.

Centers

Colloquially, health services research departments are often referred to as "shops"; in contrast to basic science research "labs." Broadly, these shops are hosted by three general types of institutions - government, academic, or non-governmental think tanks or professional societies.

Government Sponsored

- U.S. Department of Veterans Affairs Award in Health Services Research

- Institute of Medicine, U.S.-based policy research organization

University Sponsored

- Center for Surgery and Public Health, U.S. -based research institute at the Brigham and Women's Hospital (Harvard University Affiliate)

- Regenstrief Institute

- Institute for Healthcare Policy and Innovation, U.S. -based research institute at the University of Michigan (Founded in 2011, IHPI includes smaller centers focused on specific healthcare topics, such as the Center for Healthcare Outcomes & Policy

- Leonard Davis Institute of Health Economics, U.S.-based center for HSR at the University of Pennsylvania

Think Tank or Professional Society Sponsored

- Society of General Internal Medicine, U.S.-based professional organization in internal medicine research

- Commonwealth Fund, U.S.-based center for HSR

- Rand Corporation Health Division, U.S.-based center for HSR

Canada

Several government, academic and non-government agencies conduct or sponsor health services research, notably the Canadian Institute for Health Information and the Canadian Institutes of Health Research (i.e. the third pillar: "research respecting health systems and services").

Others include the Institute for Clinical Evaluative Sciences (ICES) in Toronto, and the Canadian Collaborative Study of Hip Fractures.

Denmark

Data Availability

Several registries are available for research use, such as Danish Twin Register or Danish Cancer Register.

France

Public Health Research Laboratory.

HeSPeR (Health Services and Performance Research), Université Claude Bernard Lyon 1

References

- Centers for Medicare & Medicaid Services. Fact sheet. Completion of Phase I of Medicare Health Support Program. 2008-01-28. Retrieved 2008-12-07

- White F (2015). "Primary health care and public health: foundations of universal health systems". Med Princ Pract. 24: 103–116. doi:10.1159/000370197

- Frenk J (2010). "The global health system: strengthening national health systems as the next step for global progress". PLoS Med. 7: e1000089. PMC 2797599 . PMID 20069038. doi:10.1371/journal.pmed.1000089

- Kaser, Michael (1976). "The USSR". Health care in the Soviet Union and Eastern Europe. Boulder, Colo.: Westview Press. pp. 38–39, 43. ISBN 0-89158-604-0

- "Mortality amenable to health care" Nolte, Ellen. "Variations in Amenable Mortality—Trends in 16 High-Income Nations". Commonwealth Fund. Retrieved 10 February 2012

- Kahn, James (2014). "Billing and insurance-related administrative costs in US healthcare". BMC Health Services Research. 14: 556. doi:10.1186/s12913-014-0556-7

- Handler A, Issel M, Turnock B. A conceptual framework to measure performance of the public health system. American Journal of Public Health, 2001, 91(8): 1235–39

- Collen, Morris F. A History of Medical Informatics in the United States, 1950 to 1990. Bethesda, MD: American Medical Informatics Association. ISBN 0964774305

- Kao-Ping Chua; Flávio Casoy (June 16, 2007). "Single Payer 101". American Medical Student Association. Retrieved 20 May 2014

- Carroll AE, Ackerman RT (April 2008). "Support for National Health Insurance among U.S. Physicians: 5 years later". Ann. Intern. Med. 148 (7): 566–67. PMID 18378959. doi:10.7326/0003-4819-148-7-200804010-00026

- Wall Street Journal-NBC poll: Michael McQueen, "Voters, sick of the current health-care systems, want federal government to prescribe remedy," Wall Street Journal, June 28, 1991

- David E. Kelley, "A Life of One's Own: Individual Rights and the Welfare State." Cato Institute, October 1998, ISBN 1-882577-70-1

- "The California Single-Payer Debate, The Defeat of Proposition 186 – Kaiser Family Foundation". Kff.org. Retrieved November 20, 2011

- "Universal health insurance coverage for 1.3 billion people: What accounts for China's success?". Health Policy. 119: 1145–1152. doi:10.1016/j.healthpol.2015.07.008

- O'donoghue, John; Herbert, John (2012). "Data management within mHealth environments: Patient sensors, mobile devices, and databases". Journal of Data and Information Quality (JDIQ). 4 (1): 5

- Miller RL; DK Benjamin; DC North (2003). The Economics of Public Issues (13th ed.). Boston: Addison-Wesley. ISBN 0321118731

- Greengard, Samuel (1 February 2013). "A New Model for Healthcare" (PDF). Communications of the ACM. 56 (2): 1719. doi:10.1145/2408776.2408783. Retrieved 12 February 2013

- American Society of Health-System Pharmacists (2007). "ASHP statement on the pharmacist's role in informatics". American Journal of Health-System Pharmacy. 64 (2): 200–203. doi:10.2146/ajhp060364

Permissions

Index

www.ingramcontent.com/pod-product-compliance
Lightning Source LLC
Chambersburg PA
CBHW082012190326
41458CB00010B/3162